H pylori-Associated Gastrointestinal Diseases®

Third Edition

Kathleen Graham-Lomax, MD
Research Scientist, Gastroenterology

David Y. Graham, MD
Chief, Gastroenterology Section
VA Medical Center, Houston, Texas

Professor of Medicine
Baylor College of Medicine,
Houston, Texas

Published by Handbooks in Health Care Co.
Newtown, Pennsylvania, USA

International Standard Book Number: 1-931981-49-3

Library of Congress Catalog Card Number: 2005921979

Table of Contents

This book has been prepared and is presented as a service to the medical community. The information provided reflects the knowledge, experience, and personal opinions of Kathleen Graham-Lomax, MD, Research Scientist, Short Hills, New Jersey, and David Y. Graham, MD, Professor of Medicine, Baylor College of Medicine, Houston, Texas, and Chief, Gastroenterology Section, Veterans Affairs Medical Center, Houston.

This book is not intended to replace or to be used as a substitute for the complete prescribing information prepared by each manufacturer for each drug. Because of possible variations in drug indications, in dosage information, in newly described toxicities, in drug/drug interactions, and in other items of importance, reference to such complete prescribing information is definitely recommended before any of the drugs discussed are used or prescribed.

Acknowledgments

Dr. David Y. Graham has received recent research support or honoraria for speaking engagements from AstraZeneca, Check Med, Enteric Products Inc, Meretek, Otsuka, TAP, Prometheus, Takeda, Wyeth-Ayerst, and Pharmacia. In addition, Dr. Graham is a consultant for Meretek and Otsuka. Kathleen Graham-Lomax, MD, is currently employed by Eisai Inc; no Eisai funds were used in the creation of this book.

Chapter 1

Introduction

*H**elicobacter pylori* infection is now accepted as the most common cause of gastritis and is etiologically involved in gastric ulcer, duodenal ulcer, gastric adenocarcinoma, and primary gastric B-cell lymphoma. *H pylori* infection may also play a role in some cases of nonulcer dyspepsia. *H pylori*-related diseases are among the most prevalent in the world. Thus, all physicians should be knowledgeable about the infection, its diagnosis, and management.

Helicobacter pylori and Peptic Ulcer Disease

Peptic ulcer disease is very common worldwide. Until recently, the lifetime risk of a resident of a Western nation experiencing peptic disease was approximately 10%.[1] *H pylori* is the primary cause of peptic ulcer, and, because only a proportion of the population is infected, the risk in those with *H pylori* infection is higher than in the overall population, about one in six (16%). The annual incidence of symptomatic peptic ulcer disease in the United States is 2%, with more than 500,000 new diagnoses each year and 4 million recurrences of previously identified peptic ulcers. Given these large numbers, it is not surprising that the cost to society of peptic disease is huge in terms of lost productivity and direct morbidity and mortality. For example, each year 1% to 2% of patients suffering from peptic disease will experience a major, life-threatening complication such as hemorrhage, gastric outlet obstruction, or perforation.[2] The mortality from upper gastrointestinal hemorrhage alone approaches 10%, and patients who survive a major complication are at higher risk (approximately 1% to 2% per month) for developing another life-threatening complication.

The understanding of peptic disease has shifted dramatically in the last two decades, after clinical investigation proved that *H pylori* is significant in the pathogenesis of peptic ulcer disease. Whereas peptic disease once was considered an incurable, chronic condition characterized by symptomatic episodes interspersed with symptom-free intervals, the ability to successfully treat *H pylori* infection proved that peptic disease was curable. For the first time, medical therapy was able to break the cycle of repeated episodes, as well as eliminate the risk of life-threatening complications. The therapy for this common infection is now straightforward, and diagnosis and therapy can be easily managed by a primary care provider.

Bacteria in the Stomach

Until the recent explosion of interest in *H pylori*, studies of bacteria in the stomach were usually conducted on the sidelines of medical research. Despite the 'fringe' nature of these investigations, research on the presence of bacteria in the stomach has a long and rich history. In 1893, Bizzozero reported the presence of spirochetal bacteria in canine gastric tissue; similar findings were reported by Salomon in 1896. In 1906, Balfour described spirochetes in gastric ulcers of monkeys and dogs and, in the same year, Krienitz reported similar-appearing organisms in human gastric carcinoma tissue. In the mid-1970s, Steer et al refocused attention on the presence of spiral bacteria in the stomach and their association with inflammation.[3] Unfortunately, they were unable to grow the organism in the laboratory. J. Robin Warren, a pathologist from Perth, Australia, made the critical observation that these organisms looked like *Campylobacter*. Methods to grow *Campylobacter jejuni* in the laboratory had recently been

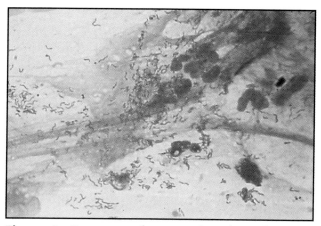

Figure 1: Gram stain of a smear from the surface of a gastric biopsy showing many gram-negative bacteria and polymorphonuclear leukocytes typical of *Helicobacter pylori* infection.

developed, and Barry Marshall, while working in the laboratory of Stewart Goodwin, was able to cultivate the bacterium now known as *H pylori*.[4]

In a 1983 letter to *Lancet*,[5] Warren and Marshall proposed a link between *H pylori* infection and peptic ulcer disease and gastric cancer. Marshall subsequently inoculated himself with a culture broth containing more than 1 billion organisms, to address whether the bacterium was a pathogen or a commensal that colonizes inflamed gastric mucosa. He developed acute gastritis within 8 days, confirming that *H pylori* causes gastritis.[6] Self-inoculation was also done by Morris, further confirming that *H pylori* is a pathogen.[7]

By the time *H pylori* was isolated, gastritis had been a target of investigation for more than 50 years. Gastritis was already associated with peptic ulcer disease, gastric cancer, and gastric lymphoma. The initial question was

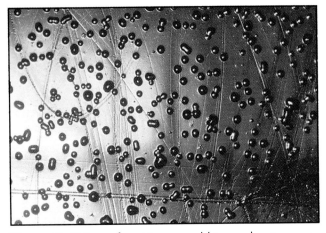

Figure 2: Culture of gastric mucosal biopsy showing many tiny, smooth, translucent colonies typical of *Helicobacter pylori*.

whether these gastritis associations could be attributed to *H pylori*. Had the cause of these diseases been discovered? The answer to both questions is yes.

The Organism

H pylori is a gram-negative rod measuring 0.6 x 3.5 microns (Figure 1). In fresh cultures, the organism is spiral-shaped, although in older cultures it can become spherical. The organism is highly motile; its sheathed, unipolar flagella lend it a darting corkscrew motion. *H pylori* is microaerophilic. Initial isolation conditions require an enriched medium, an atmosphere with reduced oxygen, ~10% CO_2, and an optimum temperature of 37°C. Growth is slow, with small (~1 mm), smooth, translucent colonies appearing after 3 days (Figure 2). Because of the slow growth, cultures should not be discarded before 14 days. The typical success rate for culture is 75% to 100%, depending on the experience of the laboratory.

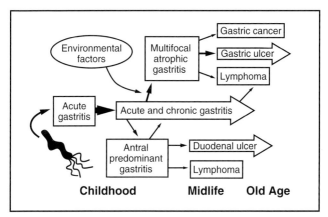

Figure 3: The potential outcomes of *Helicobacter pylori* infection. The infection is generally acquired in childhood, and most individuals go through life with asymptomatic gradual destruction of their stomach because of active chronic gastritis. About one in six people develops peptic ulcer, and, in the United States, the lifetime risk of gastric cancer is 1% to 3%. Environmental factors such as diet and standard of living are important in determining which pathway is prevalent in a country or area.

The spiral *H pylori* organism was initially named *Campylobacter pyloridis* because of structural similarities to other *Campylobacter* species. However, *'pyloridis'* is an incorrect Latin term, and, in 1987, the species name was changed to *'pylori'*. Finally, in 1989, when it became clear that *H pylori* was not a member of the genus *Campylobacter*, the genus name was changed to *Helicobacter* to reflect its distinct functional and enzymatic properties.

Importance of *Helicobacter pylori* Infection

Although most *H pylori* infections are asymptomatic, the infection is not benign (Figure 3). *H pylori* infection is a transmissible bacterial infection of the gastric mucosal surface that causes progressive damage to the gastric mucosa, with eventual impairment of gastric function. The risk of asymptomatic *H pylori* infection to the individual and to society is at least as great as that posed by asymptomatic syphilis or asymptomatic tuberculosis.[2] One significant difference between *H pylori* and those other major pathogens is that *H pylori* is always active and always transmissible. In the United States, the presence of *H pylori* infection carries a lifetime risk of peptic ulcer of at least 16%, and a 1% to 3% risk of gastric cancer. Infected individuals remain a risk to the community because the infection can be transmitted.

This book is designed to provide the practitioner with a better understanding of *H pylori*: its epidemiology, role in disease, diagnosis, and treatment. The ultimate elimination of *H pylori* would remarkably reduce suffering worldwide. *H pylori* infection is a serious public health problem, and its presence justifies treatment. The question is not whom to treat, but whom to test. If the tools were available, we would recommend screening the population for *H pylori* infection, with the goal of preventing all *H pylori*-related diseases.[8] The eventual goal should be to eliminate *H pylori* from the face of the earth, as smallpox was eliminated.

References

1. Spechler SJ: Peptic ulcer disease and its complications. In: Feldman M, Friedman LS, Sleisenger MH, eds. *Sleisenger and Fordtran's Gastrointestinal and Liver Disease,* 7th ed. Philadelphia, WB Saunders, 2002, pp 747-781.

2. Graham DY: Can therapy ever be denied for *Helicobacter pylori* infection? *Gastroenterology* 1997;113:S113-S117.

3. Steer HW, Colin-Jones DG: Mucosal changes in gastric ulceration and their response to carbenoxolone sodium. *Gut* 1975; 16:590-597.

4. Goodwin CS: *Helicobacter pylori*: 10th anniversary of its culture in April 1982. *Gut* 1993;34:293-294.

5.   Marshall BJ, Warren JR: Unidentified curved bacilli in the stomach of patients with gastritis and peptic ulceration. *Lancet* 1984;1:1311-1315.

6.   Marshall BJ, Armstrong JA, McGechie DB, et al: Attempt to fulfill Koch's postulates for pyloric *Campylobacter. Med J Aust* 1985;142:436-439.

7.   Morris A, Nicholson G: Ingestion of *Campylobacter pyloridis* causes gastritis and raised fasting gastric pH. *Am J Gastroenterol* 1987;82:192-199.

8.   Rabeneck L, Graham DY: *Helicobacter pylori*: when to test, when to treat. *Ann Intern Med* 1997;126:315-316.

Chapter **2**

Epidemiology

*H*elicobacter pylori* infects more than half the people in the world. The prevalence of the infection varies among countries and among different groups within the same country. The highest rates of infection are associated with low socioeconomic status, crowding, poor sanitation, and unclean water supplies.[1] In the United States, approximately 35% of adults are infected. However, the prevalence of infection is lower in the middle-class white population, higher in minority groups, and typically more than 80% in immigrants from developing countries.

Prevalence

H pylori infection is typically acquired in childhood. The prevalence of the infection at age 20 provides a reasonable estimate of the frequency of infection in that birth cohort throughout the remainder of their lives. In adults, the frequency of acquiring the infection is about 0.5% a year. In developed countries, the rate of acquisition of the infection is now less than the rate of loss of the infection, probably as a consequence of the use of antibiotics for a different medical problem (eg, respiratory or urinary tract infections). Thus, overall, the prevalence of *H pylori* infection is decreasing among all birth cohorts. Nonetheless, the indigent and socially disadvantaged populations in the United States still have a relatively high rate of acquisition and, along with immigrants, remain as a reservoir in the population.

Age is the most important variable related to the prevalence of infection. People born before 1950 have a notably higher rate of infection than people born later. For example, roughly half the people older than 60 years are infected, compared with 8% to 20% of those younger than 40 years. This rising infection prevalence with age is largely apparent, rather than real, reflecting a continuing overall decline in the prevalence of *H pylori* infection. Because the infection is typically acquired in childhood and is lifelong, the high proportion of older individuals (eg, age 60) who are infected is the long-term result of infection in childhood when standards of living were lower. The prevalence will decrease as current 40-year-olds, with their lower rate of infection, reach age 60, a birth cohort phenomenon (Figure 1).

Children in developing nations between the ages of 2 years and 8 years acquire the infection at a rate of about 10% a year, whereas children in the United States become infected at a rate of less than 1% a year. This significant difference in the rate of childhood acquisition is responsible for the differences in epidemiology between developed and developing countries (Figure 2).

Socioeconomic differences are the most important predictor of the prevalence of infection in any group. Higher standards of living, higher levels of education, and better sanitation correlate with lower prevalence of infection.[1] In the United States and other countries with modern sanitation and clean water supplies, the rate of acquisition has been falling since at least 1950. The rate of infection in those with several generations of high socioeconomic status is between 8% and 15%.[2] This is probably the lowest the prevalence will spontaneously fall until eradication or vaccination programs are instituted.

Helicobacter pylori Prevalence in Different Ethnic Groups

The prevalence of *H pylori* infection varies among nations, with developed, Western nations exhibiting lower rates of infection than developing countries. Even within West-

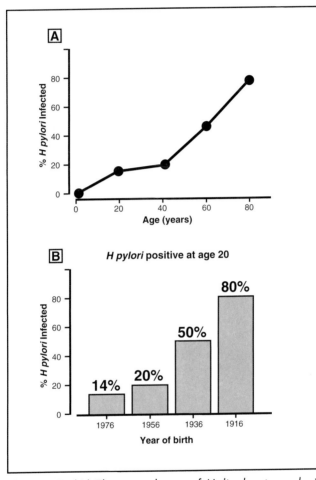

Figure 1: (A) The prevalence of *Helicobacter pylori* infection in a hypothetical US population, resulting from different rates of acquisition of infection in childhood associated with improvements in standards of living over the last century. (B) At age 20, the different birth cohorts had different prevalences of *H pylori* infection,

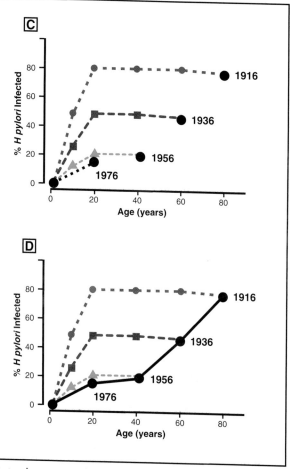

and, in this example, the prevalence at age 20 is the prevalence of infection for that birth cohort throughout life. (C) The data from (B) are plotted to show the prevalences for the different birth cohorts. (D) When the current prevalences for the different birth cohorts are joined, the current prevalence curve is reconstituted.

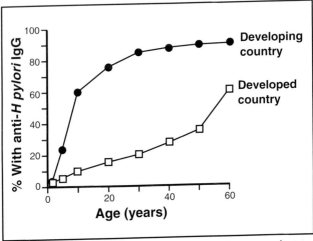

Figure 2: Rate of acquisition of *Helicobacter pylori* infection in developing and developed countries. By adulthood, most individuals living in developing countries have acquired *H pylori* infection.

ern nations, the rate of infection varies with ethnicity and race. In the United States, whites have a lower prevalence of *H pylori* infection than do blacks or Hispanics. For example, in the metropolitan Houston area, the prevalence of *H pylori* infection in blacks and Hispanics is twice that of the age-adjusted white population[3,4] (Figure 3). The difference in prevalence remained when differences in the following were controlled: income, educational level, current socioeconomic status, housing type, and use of tobacco and alcohol. Race was shown not to be the determining factor because, despite different rates of infection for whites and blacks, Hispanics (an ethnic group independent of race) had a rate of infection equal to that of blacks. When differences in socioeconomic status during *childhood* were included in the model, the differences in prevalence among the various

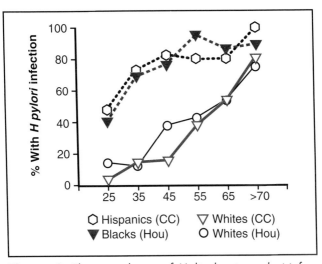

Figure 3: The prevalence of *Helicobacter pylori* infection in different populations in Houston and Corpus Christi, Texas. The prevalence of *H pylori* infection in the general population of asymptomatic non-Hispanic blacks or Hispanics was about twice that of asymptomatic whites.

groups disappeared, confirming that childhood is the critical period for acquisition of this typically lifelong infection.[5] Thus, the prevalence of *H pylori* in any group of adults reflects the rate of acquisition in childhood (Figure 4).

Genetic Factors

Although genetic factors were not an important explanation for the differences among racial or ethnic groups, genetic factors are important in determining the bacterium-host interaction and outcome of the infection.[6,7] Genetic influences are best demonstrated in studies comparing outcomes in twins raised together with those in twins separated at or near birth. This allows for comparison of the outcome

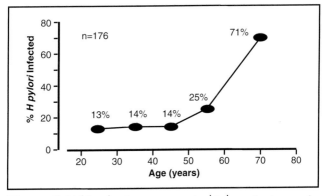

Figure 4: White dentists represent a high socioeconomic group and have a uniformly low rate until the effect of the birth cohorts of those over 65 becomes evident. Data derived from Malaty et al, *Am J Gastroenterol* 1992;87: 1728-1731.

(ie, infection or not) in monozygotic twins, who share the same genes, with that in dizygotic twins, who are genetically different. The importance of environmental factors is seen in the differences in prevalence between those reared apart compared with those reared together. Such studies have shown that monozygotic twins reared apart have concordance rates for *H pylori* infection that are much higher than those for dizygotic twins reared apart. The correlation coefficient (a measure of the influence of heritability on the prevalence of infection) was high (0.66). The range of this coefficient is between 0 and 1.[6,7] The major conclusions are that genetics are significant in acquisition of the infection, but environmental factors are also important. When the effect of socioeconomic class was investigated by studying twins raised apart in families of different economic circumstances, childhood socioeconomic status was found to have a strong influence on acquisition of *H pylori* infection.

Family Studies

Transmissibility of the infection is emphasized by several studies showing that any activity that brings together infected and uninfected individuals in situations where sanitation may be compromised is associated with a high prevalence of *H pylori* infection. For example, living in crowded circumstances in childhood has repeatedly been shown to be an epidemiologic link to risk of acquisition of the infection. Multiple studies have demonstrated an association between the number of children in the household and the risk that adult family members will acquire the infection. Studies of asymptomatic families showed that if the index case (one of the parents randomly chosen before the results of *H pylori* status were known) had *H pylori* infection, the other members of the family were likely to be infected (Figure 5). If the index parent was not infected, other members of the household were also unlikely to have *H pylori* infection. The primary source of infection within a family probably varies depending on which parent has the most contact with the children. The fact that the prevalence of *H pylori* infection in the spouse, who is genetically unrelated to the other spouse, and in the children could be predicted by the *H pylori* status of the index case is consistent with the notion that the environment is the most important factor in acquisition of *H pylori* infection. The results in families with children contrast markedly to studies of infertile couples, in which the data show little tendency for transmission from one spouse to the other.[8] Finally, although *H pylori* can be found in dental plaque, no data support kissing or sexual activity as a means of transmission. Also, no data support transmission by pets.

Clues Regarding Transmission

South Korea has undergone a huge change in its economic fortunes in the last several decades, altering itself from an underdeveloped nation to a fully industrialized

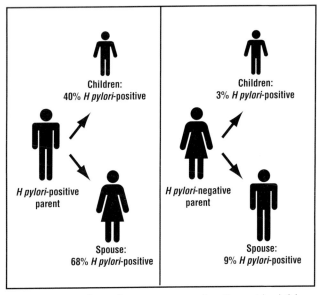

Figure 5: Studies of asymptomatic families with children found that if the randomly selected index case (either parent) were infected, the other family members had a much greater likelihood of being infected than if the index case were uninfected. Data from Malaty et al, *Scand J Gastroenterol* 1991;26:927-932.

country. This economic transformation makes Korea a particularly apt location to study the effects of socioeconomic differences on the acquisition of *H pylori* infection. Korean adults have a very high rate of infection, equivalent to rates in developing nations, reflecting the living conditions during their childhood. However, Korean children from high socioeconomic-status families had much lower prevalence rates (22%) than did children in developing nations or children of Koreans with lower socioeconomic status[9] (Figure 6). As in other countries, social class was

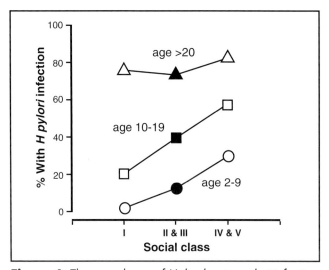

Figure 6: The prevalence of *Helicobacter pylori* infection in children and young adults in Korea. The prevalence increased with age and was inversely related to socioeconomic status. Socioeconomic class I is the highest. Data from Malaty et al, *Am J Epidemiol* 1996;143:257-262.

inversely related to prevalence of *H pylori*. Most Korean adults are infected, yet children from higher socioeconomic-status parents are becoming infected at a markedly lower rate than other socioeconomic classes, suggesting that it is possible to break the pattern of transmission. The behavior modification or mechanism resulting in the reduced rate of transmission remains unclear and is one of the important questions for further research.

Studies in relatively economically homogenous populations in China and Russia confirm that density of living is an important factor associated with risk of infection. This link between crowding and risk of infection supports the hypothesis that person-to-person transmission occurs but does not provide clues to how. Unclean water supplies in Peru and fresh vegetables grown using human wastes for fertilizer in Chile have been associated with acquisition of *H pylori* infection.[1,9] Waterborne sources of *H pylori* infection are important in some developing countries, especially those with known defective water delivery systems, but are not significant in transmission of the infection in developed countries or among populations where boiling water before consumption is routine.

Most studies suggest a fecal-oral mode of transmission, although some investigators support an oral-oral mode of transmission. *H pylori* can reach the mouth via reflux of gastric contents. While *H pylori* can be found in dental plaque, dental workers are not at increased risk to develop the infection. In addition, the lack of transmission between childless couples suggests that oral-oral transmission (eg, kissing) is unlikely to be important in transmission between adults. This, of course, does not exclude 'spitty babies' as a source of transmission within families. This would be categorized as gastric-oral and would be akin to the increased risk seen in gastroenterologists and endoscopy nurses who work with gastric secretions. Nurses in one study had a 39% rate of seropositivity compared with 26% in age-matched controls.[10] The source of *H pylori* infection in nurses could be fecal-oral or gastric-oral, associated with handling of nasogastric tubes or endoscopes.

H pylori infection clusters in families with small children, suggesting that the presence of infants and small children somehow acts as an amplifier, vector, or facilitator of intrafamily transmission.[11] Iatrogenic spread of *H pylori* infection also has been documented. The exact route of transmission remains unclear. Data support fecal-oral and oral-oral paths; both probably are correct. We consider *H pylori* to be 'opportunistic' in that it takes advantage of any break in sanitation that allows it to enter the stomach of an uninfected host; therefore, a wide variety

Table 1: Risk Factors for
Helicobacter pylori **Infection**

- Birth in a developing country
- Low socioeconomic status
- Crowded living conditions
- Large families
- Unsanitary living conditions
- Unclean food or water
- Presence of infants in the home
- Exposure to gastric contents of infected individuals
    - (a) gastrointestinal endoscopists
    - (b) nurses

of circumstances can result in a route of transmission (Table 1). Studies are needed to identify simple measures (eg, hand washing) or behaviors that can be modified in the family or day-care center to reduce or eliminate transmission. Unfortunately, these studies may need to be repeated in different populations because the primary mode of transmission may vary depending on cultural practices, especially as they relate to household hygiene.

H pylori can be differentiated by comparing the genotypes of the strains. This technique allows one to compare the type of *H pylori* with the geographic origin of the individual or group. For example, we have shown that *H pylori* from Native Americans has many characteristics found only among *H pylori* strains from Asia, confirming that *H pylori* entered the Americas before Columbus. Even within the Americas, there are differences suggesting that native populations in South America predated those currently living in Alaska. Some Native Alaskans were found to have *H pylori* strains similar to those currently found in Kazakhstan, suggesting that they arrived later and from Central Asia. Studies within different ethnic groups showed that ethnic groups in which there is limited intermarriage tended to retain the strains characteristic of the place of origin of their ethnic group such that the Hispanic population had strains similar to those found among current inhabitants of the Iberian peninsula. Those whose ancestors came to the United States from Northern Europe had 'Northern European' strains.[12] Within Hispanic families, where the mother is typically the primary caregiver, the *H pylori* from the children were the same as those of the mother. Studies using such molecular epidemiologic techniques are needed to help trace the primary patterns of transmission within different cultures so that effective prevention strategies can be developed. The development of minimally invasive techniques to obtain *H pylori* will foster such studies, and the results are eagerly awaited.

References

1.   Breuer T, Malaty HM, Graham DY: The epidemiology of *H pylori*-associated gastroduodenal diseases. In: Ernst PB, Michetti P, Smith PD, eds. *The Immunobiology of H pylori: From Pathogenesis to Prevention*. Philadelphia, Lippincott-Raven, 1997, pp 1-14.

2.   Malaty HM, Evans DJ Jr, Abramovitch K, et al: *Helicobacter pylori* infection in dental workers: a seroepidemiology study. *Am J Gastroenterol* 1992;87:1728-1731.

3.   Graham DY, Malaty HM, Evans DG, et al: Epidemiology of *Helicobacter pylori* in an asymptomatic population in the United States. Effect of age, race, and socioeconomic status. *Gastroenterology* 1991;100:1495-1501.

4.   Malaty HM, Evans DG, Evans DJ Jr, et al: *Helicobacter pylori* in Hispanics: comparison with blacks and whites of similar age and socioeconomic class. *Gastroenterology* 1992;103:813-816.

5.   Malaty HM, Graham DY: Importance of childhood socioeconomic status on the current prevalence of *Helicobacter pylori* infection. *Gut* 1994;35:742-745.

6.   Go MF, Graham DY: Determinants of clinical outcome of *H pylori* infection: duodenal ulcer. In: Hunt RH, Tytgat GN, eds. *Helicobacter pylori*: *Basic Mechanisms to Clinical Cure*. Dordrecht, Netherlands, Kluwer Academic Publishers, 1994, pp 421-428.

7.   Graham DY, Malaty HM, Go MF: Are there susceptible hosts to *Helicobacter pylori* infection? *Scand J Gastroenterol Suppl* 1994;205:6-10.

8.   Perez-Perez GI, Witkin SS, Decker MD, et al: Seroprevalence of *Helicobacter pylori* infection in couples. *J Clin Microbiol* 1991;29:642-644.

9.   Malaty HM, Kim JG, Kim SD, et al: Prevalence of *Helicobacter pylori* infection in Korean children: inverse relation to socioeconomic status despite a uniformly high prevalence in adults. *Am J Epidemiol* 1996;143:257-262.

10.   Wilhoite SL, Ferguson DA Jr, Soike DR, et al: Increased prevalence of *Helicobacter pylori* antibodies among nurses. *Arch Intern Med* 1993;153:708-712.

11.   Graham DY, Klein PD, Evans DG, et al: *Helicobacter pylori*: epidemiology, relationship to gastric cancer and the role of infants in transmission. *Eur J Gastroenterol Hepatol* 1992;4:S1-S6.

12.   Yamaoka Y, Malaty HM, Osato MS, et al: Conservation of *Helicobacter pylori* genotypes in different ethnic groups in Houston, Texas. *J Infect Dis* 2000;181:2083-2086.

Chapter **3**

Effect of *Helicobacter pylori* Infection on Gastroduodenal Physiology

The stomach once was viewed as a cauldron of acid, inhospitable to colonization by microorganisms. However, research has proven that many species of bacteria can call the stomach their home, chief among them *Helicobacter pylori*. *H pylori* holds a unique niche, namely, living within and beneath the mucus layer of the stomach. To fully understand the effect of colonization by *H pylori* on gastroduodenal physiology, normal physiology should first be explored.

Gastric Function

The stomach serves as the reservoir for food and initiates digestion mechanically, through grinding and mixing, and also by chemical processes. Pathogen control is an essential function of this acid-filled organ. The low pH of the stomach fluid degrades and kills most ingested microorganisms. Indeed, in the healthy stomach, many bacteria are rendered inactive in 15 minutes when the pH is 3 or less. For example, when the stomach pH is between 2 and 3, most pathogenic species of bacteria are killed within 1 hour, including *Campylobacter jejuni*, *Yersinia enterocolitica*, *Salmonella*, and *Shigella*. When the ambient gastric pH rises to 4 or 6, these organisms survive. As these results suggest, reduced acid secretion is associated with increased risk of enteric infections.

Acid Secretion

Comparative physiology studies have shown that nearly every vertebrate organism has some portion of gastric mucosa that secretes hydrochloric acid.[1] Infection by *H pylori* may result in gradual destruction of the normal gastric mucosa, causing gastric atrophy. Regulation of the acidic environment of the stomach is complex and carefully controlled. Acid secretion occurs over three phases. The cephalic phase is controlled by the vagus nerve. After vagal stimulation, cholinergic receptors are stimulated, leading to release of histamine from enterochromaffin-like cells (the most common endocrine cell in the stomach) and parietal cell stimulation. The gastric phase of acid secretion is caused by secretion of gastrin from the antrum and is down-regulated by somatostatin. The final phase, the intestinal phase, is related to the entry of nutrients into the small intestine.

Gastric Mucus

The body expends energy to generate an acidic environment in the stomach and produce the mucus coating that protects the surface epithelial layer of the stomach. Mucin is a polymeric, strongly hydrophilic, gel-forming substance that functions as a lubricant, binds microorganisms and toxins, and helps retain bicarbonate ions secreted by the surface cells to maintain a neutral environment adjacent to the epithelial surface. The mucus layer is continually worn away at the luminal surface because of interaction with acid and pepsin, and it must be constantly regenerated by the surface cells. *H pylori* primarily colonizes the stomach within and just below this mucus layer.

Helicobacter pylori Survival Strategies

H pylori is well suited to survive in this hostile environment.[2] On ingestion, the organism uses its motility (via flagella) to swim to and penetrate the mucus layer. It then can burrow to the mucosal surface, where it is protected from the intensely acidic gastric fluid. Production of ammonia by the organism's urease enzyme is important in shielding the organism from acid during its transit to the gastric mucosal surface. The importance of urease activity as a virulence factor was confirmed by experiments showing that, with only a few exceptions, urease-negative mutants were unable to colonize experimental animals.

While *H pylori* is generally not considered invasive, it can be found within epithelial cells, suggesting that an intracellular location may serve as a sanctuary for evasion of host defenses and may be responsible for the failure of topical antibiotic therapy. *H pylori* attaches selectively to the surface mucus-secreting cells of the stomach. Complex adhesin molecules mediate the attachment process and account for the organism's tissue and host specificity.[3] Attachment of *H pylori* to the mucosa results in cytoskeletal changes in the cell, with the appearance of adherence pedestals similar to those seen in enteropathogenic strains of *Escherichia coli*. The site of adherence is typically the intercellular junctions of the epithelial cells. *H pylori* has been found in any area with gastric surface cells, including areas with heterotopic gastric mucosa or with gastric metaplasia (eg, in the duodenum and even the rectum).

Virulence Factors

Many bacterial diseases can be related to specific virulence factors (eg, cholera to cholera toxin, diphtheria to diphtheria toxin). The clinical manifestations of an infectious disease often are multifactorial and influenced by prior exposure to the agent or virulence factor. For example, vaccination allows an individual to harbor *Corynebacterium diphtheriae* and not experience disease. The virulence factor is required to produce the disease (ie, no diphtheria toxin = no diphtheria). The extensive experience with disease-specific virulence factors in other bacterial infections led to an ongoing and intensive search for disease-specific virulence factors for *H pylori*. The first candidates were the vacuolating cytotoxin and a protein named CagA. CagA has subsequently been identified as a component of the *cag* pathogenicity island.[4] The initial observations were encouraging, showing a statistically significant higher frequency of CagA-positive *H pylori* in patients with duodenal ulcer, compared with patients without ulcer disease. Subsequently, an association was shown between CagA positivity and gastric cancer and the precursor lesion, atrophic gastritis.[5] This latter association caused some concern because the two diseases (gastric cancer and duodenal ulcer disease) are believed to be mutually exclusive.[6] Not all studies have confirmed the CagA-disease associations, and a number of recent studies cast additional doubt on the association of CagA and gastric adenocarcinoma. Two of the European countries with the highest incidences of gastric cancer (Iceland and Portugal) have a low proportion of CagA-positive strains. Furthermore, the incidence of gastric cancer continues to decrease, suggesting that if CagA-positive strains were critically important, the prevalence of CagA positivity would have fallen in parallel, and it did not. Studies from Asia and the United States also have failed to show any disease specificity associated with CagA, primarily because more than 95% of *H pylori* strains in those regions contain the virulence factor. Worldwide, at least 70% of *H pylori* strains are CagA positive. Serologic tests have been developed to detect the presence of anti-CagA antibody but typically have proven to be inaccurate, underestimating the true prevalence of the factor. There is no clinical use in attempting to identify CagA-positive *H pylori* because peptic ulcers and gastric cancer have been found to be associated with CagA-negative *H pylori*.[7,8]

Recently, a new inflammation-associated virulence factor has been identified, the *outer inflammatory protein*, or OipA.[9] OipA is one of the outer membrane proteins of *H pylori* and is involved in production of mucosal inflammation. An active OipA appears to greatly accentuate the ability of strains with the *cag* pathogenicity island to cause inflammation. *H pylori* can contain a functional or a nonfunctional OipA, and current data suggest that the presence of a functional OipA is a better predictor of a symptomatic outcome than any other virulence factor. In East Asia, probably 95% or more of *H pylori* are CagA and OipA positive. We consider these strains hypervirulent, but even they do not have a high direct linkage with ultimate presentation with a symptomatic outcome.

H pylori is a gram-negative organism, and physicians are well aware of the importance of endotoxin (lipopolysaccharide [LPS]) in disease. Studies have shown that *H pylori* LPS is particularly low in biologic activity, which probably gives the organism a survival advantage considering that the infection continues for decades. Indeed, the LPS polymers have been found to be 1,000-fold less toxic than comparative molecules from other gram-negative bacteria.[10]

H pylori is able to protect itself by evading host defenses, and much research focuses on understanding this immune evasion. The location of the organism on the luminal surface of gastric epithelial cells and in areas of low oxygen tension and low pH, as well as in places relatively inaccessible to the body's defenses, such as gastric glands and parietal cell canaliculi, may be critical in allowing the organism to survive attack by the host's immune system. *H pylori* contains superoxide dismutase and catalase, which might help protect the organism from phagocyte-derived reactive oxygen metabolites. Superoxide dismutase-deficient mutations are lethal to the bacteria, suggesting a crucial role for this enzyme in the life of the bacterium.[10]

In summary, the importance of virulence factors in other bacterial infection is largely related to acute infections. *H pylori* produces a chronic infection, and it may be important to rethink the role and consequence of putative virulence factors. The pattern and severity of inflammation are the key determinants of outcome, and these relate to host, environmental, and bacterial factors. As will be examined later, the critical environmental factors are probably dietary. Host factors may relate to genetic polymorphormisms in genes controlling the extent and severity of the inflammatory response to the infection. The important disease-associated virulence factors of the bacteria may be those that enhance inflammation, currently OipA and CagA. Integration of the three areas will be required to understand the outcome in an individual patient.

Helicobacter pylori-Induced Inflammation

Once the organism is acquired, has passed through the mucus layer, and takes up residence at the luminal surface of the stomach, an intense inflammatory response of the underlying tissue develops. The presence of *H pylori* is always associated with tissue damage and the histologic findings of an acute and a chronic gastritis. How does a luminal, 'offshore' organism induce these changes in tissue it has not directly invaded? *H pylori* infection is a bacterial infection of a mucosal surface, and it should not be surprising that an organism that attaches to and interacts with gastric epithelial cells would result in inflammation. Numerous other surface infections lead to inflammatory changes in underlying tissue (eg, acute infections such as urinary tract infections, chronic infections such as periodontal disease). The interaction of *H pylori* with the surface mucosa results in release of the proinflammatory cytokine IL-8, which leads to recruitment of polymorphonuclear cells and may begin the inflammatory process.[11] The uptake of *H pylori* into epithelial cells is sufficient reason for an inflammatory response. Gastric epithelial cells express class II molecules that may increase the inflammatory response by presenting *H pylori* antigens, leading to further cytokine release and more inflammation.

Biopsy of *H pylori*-infected gastric mucosa reveals large numbers of inflammatory cells, especially phagocytes and plasma cells (Figure 1). High levels of proinflammatory cytokines are detected, particularly TNF-α and numerous interleukins (eg, IL-6, IL-8, IL-10). Leukotriene levels are also elevated, especially leukotriene B$_4$, which is synthesized by host neutrophils and is cytotoxic to gastric epithelium.[2] This inflammatory response leads to functional changes in the stomach, depending on the involved areas of the stomach. When the inflammation is corpus-predominant, parietal cells are inhibited, leading to reduced acid secretion. Continued inflammation results in loss of parietal cells, and the reduction in acid secretion becomes permanent. Antral inflammation alters the interplay between gastrin and somatostatin secretion, affecting G cells (gastrin-secreting) and D cells (somatostatin-secreting), respectively. Specifically, gastrin secretion is abnormal in *H pylori*-infected individuals, with an exaggerated meal-stimulated release of gastrin most prominent. When the infection is cured, neutrophil infiltration of the tissue quickly resolves, with slower resolution of the chronic inflammatory cells. Meal-stimulated gastrin secretion returns to normal in parallel with the slow resolution of the monocytic infiltrates. Much research has focused on the perturbations of gastrin secretion, and the link has proven related to the effects of chronic inflammation and not attributable to a direct effect of *H pylori*.[12]

Helicobacter pylori-Induced Perturbations in Acid Secretion

H pylori-induced inflammation in the gastric corpus reduces acid secretion, probably through a cytokine-mediated mechanism (eg, IL-1).[13] This reduction in acid secretion allows the bacteria to associate with the mucosal cells, promoting inflammation and further decreasing acid secretion.[14] The nature of this interaction between *H pylori* and the mucosal cells is unclear but is likely related, in part, to the depth of bacterial penetration into the pits. It has been hypothesized that any event that reduces acid secretion potentially promotes the development (or in-

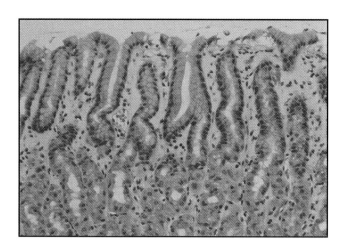

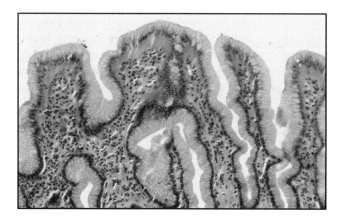

Figure 1: Photomicrograph (top) of normal stomach with a paucity of inflammatory cells. Active *Helicobacter pylori* infection (bottom) in which the gastric mucosa is actively inflamed. The mucosa is infiltrated with acute and chronic inflammatory cells, and *H pylori* is seen on the surface.

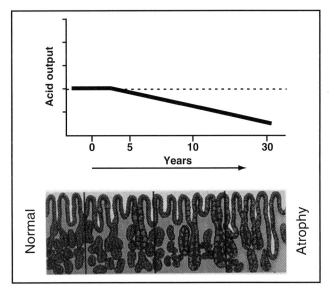

Figure 2: The natural history of *Helicobacter pylori* gastritis is gradual destruction of the gastric mucosal architecture with loss of glands and reduction in acid secretion, leading to atrophy. The rate of progress varies among individuals. Patients with duodenal ulcer have mild corpus gastritis, and acid secretion remains high for decades.

crease) of corpus gastritis, which in turn leads to an increase in the distribution of atrophic gastritis[14] (Figure 2).

Because the infection is most likely acquired in childhood, events in childhood are most important in determining outcome.[14] In childhood, malnutrition, vitamin deficiency, a diet poor in fresh fruits and vegetables, or the development of any of a number of childhood infectious diseases transiently reduces acid secretion and, if the child is already infected with *H pylori*, may allow for development of corpus gastritis and begin the spiral toward development of atrophic gastritis. In contrast, *H pylori*-infected children with diets adequate in fresh fruits and vegetables (which promote a healthy corpus mucosa) are more likely to have gastritis limited to the antrum, to have minimal corpus gastritis, and to be at risk for development of peptic ulcer instead of gastric cancer.

It should become obvious that the simple models have given way to more complex ones (Figure 3). These were required to fit the data available about the relative frequencies of infection and *H pylori*-related diseases (eg, different frequencies of cancer among various regions of Colombia or Japan despite the same frequency of *H pylori* infection). The search for a duodenal ulcer-specific dysregulation in acid secretion, or for an *H pylori*-induced duodenal dysregulation in acid secretion, has been fruitless. After many false starts (eg, hypotheses suggesting a critical role for exaggerated meal-stimulated gastrin release or exaggerated gastrin-releasing peptide-induced acid secretion), it became clear that no duodenal ulcer-specific dysregulations occur in acid secretion, and the initial optimism was related to incomplete studies or incomplete understanding of normal gastric physiology. The current hypothesis that links *H pylori* and duodenal ulcer disease is related to the inhibition of growth of *H pylori* by bile and the precipitation of bile acids by acid[14,15] (Figure 3). Thus, any event that directly or indirectly increases the duodenal acid load by reducing the ability of the duodenum to neutralize acid (eg, smoking does both) would be associated with an increased risk of development of *H pylori*-associated duodenal ulcer disease (Table 1). The presence of *H pylori* infection in the duodenal bulb and the associated inflammation, and the presence of junctional epithelium between the inflamed gastric metaplasia and the villous epithelium, may weaken the mucosa and compromise the repair processes such that chronic ulcer disease develops.[16]

Gastritis also is strongly associated with peptic ulcer disease. This association extends back more than 70 years.

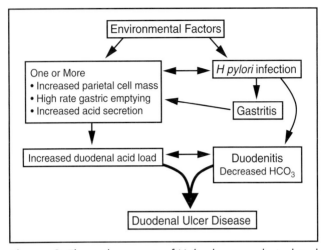

Figure 3: The pathogenesis of *Helicobacter pylori*-related duodenal ulcer disease requires *H pylori* infection of gastric metaplasia in the duodenal bulb. Because *H pylori* is inhibited by bile acids, a sufficient duodenal acid load is needed to precipitate the bile salts from the luminal contents. The duodenal acid load is increased by factors that increase delivery of acid to the duodenum and by factors that reduce the ability of the duodenum to produce bicarbonate to neutralize the acid entering it.

The comments of Faber are interesting and instructive. He summarized available research in 1927, noting the association of duodenal ulcer with antral predominant gastritis. Faber suggested that gastritis was finally ready to assume its proper place in research on the etiology of peptic ulcer.[17] He observed that studies of gastric physiology had often overlooked gastritis, and hoped that this trend was over. He would be disappointed for another 60 years.

Research on the role of gastritis in peptic ulcer disease remained a backwater area and was overshadowed by the

Table 1: Factors Increasing the Duodenal Acid Load

Increased acid secretion

- Large parietal cell mass
- Smoking
- Stress
- Impaired down-regulation of acid secretion (*H pylori* infection)

Decreased duodenal bicarbonate secretion

- *H pylori* infection (inflammation)
- Smoking

rapid advances in the understanding of the physiology of gastric acid and pepsin secretion. The development of H_2-receptor antagonists was associated with a major leap forward in the understanding of acid secretion, and the 1970s and 1980s were a time of rapid advances in understanding normal and abnormal gastric function in duodenal ulcer disease. Research focused on discovery of a perturbation in gastric physiology that was responsible for development of duodenal ulcer disease. The new technique of radioimmunoassay allowed for measurement of gastrin concentrations and correlation with acid secretion. Intragastric titration and perfusion techniques allowed meal-stimulated acid secretion to be directly measured in health and disease. The results of these experiments greatly increased our knowledge of the normal and abnormal regulation of acid secretion but failed to identify an ulcer-specific dysregulation in acid secretion.[18] Increasingly, it began to appear that no ulcer-specific dysregulation was present, which opened the road to new concepts in the pathogenesis of ulcer disease. The discovery of *H pylori* provided a unifying factor that has allowed for progress and new understandings of gastric physiology and new hypotheses about the pathogenesis of gastroduodenal diseases.

One key to this better understanding is the recognition that the status of the gastric corpus mucosa is critical. Inflammation in the corpus reversibly inhibits acid secretion.[19] Loss of parietal cells (eg, atrophy) probably leads to an irreversible reduction in acid secretion. Future studies must provide data on the status of the corpus mucosa, use maximum stimuli for acid secretion (eg, pentagastrin and not gastrin-releasing peptide), and be repeated after the infection is cured. We now have a general framework for the perturbations in gastric physiology related to *H pylori* infection. These insights should be extended to the mechanisms at the cellular and molecular levels, and new therapies possibly developed based on insights over the next decade. Our understanding has increased such that it is possible to predict the effect of *H pylori* infection on acid secretion.

References

1.   Sachs G, Hersey SJ, Pounder RE, et al: Gastric secretion. In: Gustavsson S, Kumar D, Graham DY, eds. *The Stomach.* New York, Churchill Livingstone, 1992, pp 41-79.

2.   Dunn BE: Pathogenic mechanisms of *Helicobacter pylori. Gastroenterol Clin North Am* 1993;22:43-57.

3.   Doig P, Trust TJ: The molecular basis for *H pylori* adherence and colonization. In: Ernst PB, Michetti P, Smith PD, eds. *The Immunobiology of H pylori: From Pathogenesis to Prevention.* Philadelphia, Lippincott-Raven, 1997, pp 47-58.

4.   Censini S, Lange C, Xiang Z, et al: cag, a pathogenicity island of *Helicobacter pylori*, encodes type I-specific and disease-associated virulence factors. *Proc Natl Acad Sci U S A* 1996;93:14648-14653.

5.   Blaser MJ: Role of vacA and the cagA locus of *Helicobacter pylori* in human disease. *Aliment Pharmacol Ther* 1996;10:73-77.

6.   Graham DY, Go MF, Genta RM: *Helicobacter pylori*, duodenal ulcer, gastric cancer: tunnel vision or blinders? *Ann Med* 1995;27:589-594.

7.   Miehlke S, Bayerdorffer E, Graham DY: Treatment of *Helicobacter pylori* infection. *Semin Gastrointest Dis* 2001;12:167-179.

8. Graham DY, Qureshi WA: Markers of infection. In: Mobley HL, Mendz GL, Hazell SL, eds. *Helicobacter pylori*: *Physiology and Genetics*. Washington, DC, ASM Press, 2001, pp 499-510.

9. Yamaoka Y, Kwon DH, Graham DY: A M(r) 34,000 proinflammatory outer membrane protein (oipA) of *Helicobacter pylori*. *Proc Natl Acad Sci U S A* 2000;97:7533-7538.

10. Ernst PB, Pecquet S: Interactions between *Helicobacter pylori* and the local mucosal immune system. *Scand J Gastroenterol Suppl* 1991;187:56-64.

11. Crabtree JE: Virulence factors of *H pylori* and their effect on chemokine production. In: Ernst PB, Michetti P, Smith PD, eds. *The Immunobiology of H pylori*: *From Pathogenesis to Prevention*. Philadelphia, Lippincott-Raven, 1997, pp 101-112.

12. Calam J: *Helicobacter pylori*, acid and gastrin. *Eur J Gastroenterol Hepatol* 1995;7:310-317.

13. Clemens J, Albert MJ, Rao M, et al: Impact of infection by *Helicobacter pylori* on the risk and severity of endemic cholera. *J Infect Dis* 1995;171:1653-1656.

14. Graham DY: *Helicobacter pylori* infection in the pathogenesis of duodenal ulcer and gastric cancer: a model. *Gastroenterology* 1997;113:1983-1991.

15. Graham DY, Genta RM, Go MF, et al: Which is the most important factor in duodenal ulcer pathogenesis: the strain of *Helicobacter pylori* or the host? In: Hunt RH, Tytgat GN, eds. *Helicobacter pylori*: *Basic Mechanisms to Clinical Cure*. Dordrecht, Netherlands, Kluwer Academic Publishers, 1996, pp 85-91.

16. Graham DY: *Campylobacter pylori* and peptic ulcer disease. *Gastroenterology* 1989;96:615-625.

17. Faber K: Chronic gastritis: its relation to achylia and ulcer. *Lancet* 1927;2:902-907.

18. Soll AH: Gastric, duodenal, and stress ulcer. In: Sleisenger M, Fordtran J, eds. *Gastrointestinal Disease*, 5th ed. Philadelphia, WB Saunders, 1993, pp 580-679.

19. Gutierrez O, Melo M, Segura AM, et al: Cure of *Helicobacter pylori* infection improves gastric acid secretion in patients with corpus gastritis. *Scand J Gastroenterol* 1997;32:664-668.

Chapter 4

Associated Diseases

*H*elicobacter pylori infects more than half the world's population. It is a major pathogen that causes gastritis and the gastritis-associated diseases peptic ulcer, gastric adenocarcinoma, and primary gastric B-cell lymphoma (Table 1). Associations between *H pylori* infection and other conditions are tenuous and speculative (Table 2).

Gastritis

The self-inoculation experiments by Marshall and Morris proved that *H pylori* infection causes gastritis. Subse-

---

**Table 1: Potential Outcomes
of *Helicobacter pylori* Infection**

- Transmission of the infection to others
- Damage to gastric structure and function (100%)
  - Development of hypochlorhydria
    or achlorhydria (~25%)
    (a) increased enteric infections
    (b) reduced absorption of iron and vitamin B_{12}
- Development of peptic ulcer (~17%)
  - Ulcer complication (~20%)
- Development of gastric adenocarcinoma (1% to 3% in the United States, 11% to 12% in Japan)
- Development of primary gastric lymphoma
- Development of nonulcer dyspepsia

Table 2: Suggested Links Poorly Supported in the Literature and Lacking Appropriate Controls

- Food allergy
- Gallstones
- Short stature
- Thyroid disease
- Chronic urticaria
- Headache
- Diabetes
- Raynaud's phenomenon

quent studies in which antimicrobial therapy resulted in healing of gastritis extended the hypothesis to include the possibility that eradication of the infection might cure, or even prevent, a number of important and prevalent gastroduodenal diseases associated with gastritis. Understanding the outlines of the epidemiology of *H pylori* infection was relatively straightforward once the connection was made between *H pylori* and gastritis. The wealth of existing data on gastritis and its associated conditions, natural history, and epidemiology then could be transferred to *H pylori* infection.[1] A number of studies rapidly confirmed that such a transfer was appropriate.

Infection with *H pylori* is universally associated with histopathologic findings of mucosal inflammation (ie, gastritis).[2,3] The severity of the gastritis may vary in different regions of the stomach and is typically most severe in the non–acid-secreting portions of the stomach, antrum, and cardia.

Normal gastric mucosa is essentially devoid of inflammatory cells. *H pylori* infection leads to infiltration of the

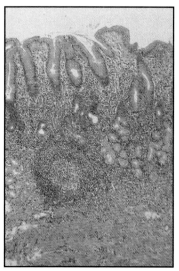

Figure 1: Photomicrograph showing large lymphoid follicle with germinal centers in *Helicobacter pylori*-infected gastric mucosa. The normal stomach is devoid of organized lymphoid structures. Finding lymphoid follicles in otherwise normal gastric mucosa suggests past *H pylori* infection.

stomach with polymorphonuclear cells (active inflammation) and with mononuclear inflammatory cells (chronic inflammation), resulting in a pattern of active-chronic gastritis. Over time, the lymphoid infiltration in the gastric mucosa, *mucosa-associated lymphoid tissue (MALT)*, becomes prominent, with lymphoid follicles becoming evident (Figure 1). Even though *H pylori* is found throughout the stomach, the inflammation is often mild, superficial, or even absent in the gastric corpus. The natural history of gastritis is extension of the inflamed area from the antrum into the corpus, resulting in a reduction in acid secretion and eventually loss of parietal cells and development of atrophy.

Risk Factor for Gastric Atrophy

Chronic gastritis is the precursor lesion for development of gastric atrophy. *H pylori* and autoimmune gastritis leading to pernicious anemia are the chief causes of gastric atrophy. Chronic *H pylori* infection may progress from

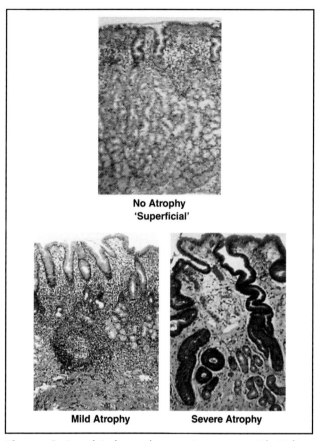

No Atrophy
'Superficial'

Mild Atrophy **Severe Atrophy**

Figure 2: Panel 1 shows the gastric mucosa with *Helico-bacter pylori*-associated inflammation without atrophy. Panels 2 and 3 show progressive loss of normal glandular elements as the disease progresses to gastric atrophy.

chronic gastritis to gastric atrophy (Figure 2). Corpus inflammation results in inhibition of acid secretion and eventual loss of normal cellular elements. This scenario is not inevitable and occurs in a subpopulation of infected adults at a rate of 1% to 2% a year.[4] The rate of progression to atrophy varies in different geographic regions related to other environmental factors; diet is probably the most important. Atrophic gastritis is the central precursor lesion in the progression from superficial gastritis to gastric cancer.

Risk of Disease

The relationship between *H pylori* and gastritis is constant and direct. Only a small proportion of those with *H pylori* infection develop clinically symptomatic outcomes such as peptic ulcer disease or gastric cancer[5] (Table 1). Most patients with *H pylori* infection develop neither. Although the reason only a proportion of those with the infection develop symptomatic disease is unclear, it also occurs in other chronic infectious diseases, such as asymptomatic syphilis or tuberculosis. In fact, the proportion with a clinical outcome is higher with *H pylori* than with either of the other two chronic infections. Factors that may be important include interaction with environmental factors, differences in host susceptibility, and virulence of the *H pylori* strain.[6]

Peptic Ulcer Disease

H pylori infection is closely linked to peptic disease. Most series show that *H pylori* infection accounts for most duodenal ulcers and approximately 70% of gastric ulcers (Figure 3). *H pylori* infection is not the only cause of peptic ulcer. Use of nonsteroidal anti-inflammatory drugs (NSAIDs) is the other major cause of peptic ulcers; in regions where the prevalence of *H pylori* infection is low, it is the most common cause. Recent studies in which the percentage of ulcers associated with *H pylori* was reported to be 'lower than expected' likely actually reflect the low *H pylori* prevalence in the population studied. For example, looking simply at the percentage of patients with duodenal ulcer and *H pylori* infection, the proportion will vary depending on the preva-

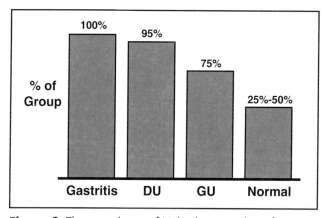

Figure 3: The prevalence of *Helicobacter pylori* infection in different diseases. DU = duodenal ulcer; GU = gastric ulcer.

lence of *H pylori* and the prevalence of other potential causes of duodenal ulcer disease.

Consider two populations, each with 100,000 individuals. One population is of lower socioeconomic status and is served by a charity hospital. The other population is upper middle class and seen by private specialists. The prevalence of *H pylori* infection in the indigent population is 80%, compared with 20% in the private patient group. Assume that the use of NSAIDs is the same in both groups (14%). Further assume that endoscopic sampling of both populations yields a point prevalence of duodenal ulcer of 1% in those with *H pylori* infection and 1% in the NSAID users. The total number of duodenal ulcers in the *H pylori*-infected population is therefore a function of the prevalence of *H pylori* and can be calculated: number of *H pylori* duodenal ulcers equals (population size) times (prevalence) times (point prevalence of duodenal ulcer).

Thus, in this hypothetical situation, 800 duodenal ulcers would be caused by *H pylori* in the indigent patients and only 200 in the private patients (100,000 x 0.8 x 0.01

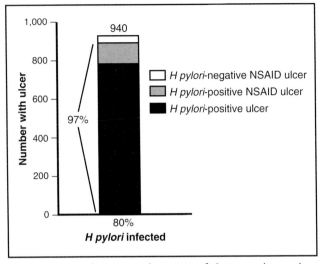

Figure 4: In this example, 80% of the population has *Helicobacter pylori* infection. Thus, 80% of ulcers from another cause would be expected to have coincidental *H pylori* infection. The prevalence of *H pylori* infection in duodenal ulcer disease would be 97%.

vs. $100,000 \times 0.2 \times 0.01$). The number of NSAID ulcers would be identical in the two populations ($100,000 \times 0.14 \times 0.01 = 140$). The proportion of patients with *H pylori* infection and duodenal ulcer in the population with a background prevalence of *H pylori* infection of 80% would be high (97%) (Figure 4), because 80% of the patients with NSAID ulcers would also have incidental *H pylori* infection. In contrast, the proportion of patients with duodenal ulcer without *H pylori* infection in the population with a low background incidence of *H pylori* infection would be high. Figure 5 illustrates that the indigent patient population would have 800 *H pylori* ulcers, 112 NSAID ulcers with incidental *H pylori* infec-

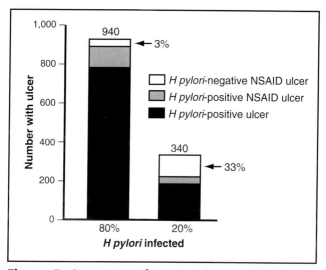

Figure 5: Comparison of two populations with the same incidence of *Helicobacter pylori* and NSAID ulcers but different background prevalence of *H pylori* infection. The proportion of *H pylori*-positive ulcers is greatly overestimated when the background prevalence of the infection is high. Conversely, it would superficially appear that *H pylori* would have a minor role in the pathogenesis of duodenal ulcer in the population with a low background prevalence. Studies that only look at percentages of a population with a disease with more than one cause can be greatly misleading.

tion, and only 28 NSAID-only ulcers. The percentage of *H pylori*-negative duodenal ulcers in the indigent patients would therefore be 3%, compared with 33% of the private patients. Importantly, the total number of ulcers in the different populations also is remarkably different, with only 340 total ulcers in the private patients compared with 940 in the group with a high background prevalence of *H pylori* infection.

Misleading conclusions can be derived from studies using only percentage data. To understand the results in any population, data are needed on the prevalence of the possible causes of ulcer, as well as the point prevalence of ulcers from any cause. This reasoning can be extended to any *H pylori*-related disease (eg, a lesser proportion of gastric cancer patients would be expected to be *H pylori* positive in a population with a low prevalence of *H pylori* infection compared with a high-prevalence population). This also explains why the proportion of patients who suffer ulcer relapse after cure of the infection may vary among different studies. A high rate of *H pylori* infection in any population can 'disguise' ulcers with another etiology, and that other etiology will become evident after the *H pylori* infection is eliminated. The prevalence of *H pylori* in the white middle and upper class US population is now in the range of 8% to 15% such that the few chronic ulcers that do occur are often not *H pylori* ulcers. As will be examined later, this has major implications with regard to making an accurate etiologic diagnosis before beginning curative therapy.

Causal Evidence

The strong link between *H pylori* and peptic ulcer, and the observation that cure of the infection results in cure of the ulcer disease, provided strong evidence that *H pylori* is etiologic in the pathogenesis of peptic ulcer disease. Researchers have considered whether Koch's postulates have been fulfilled for the hypothesis that *H pylori* causes ulcers[7]; Howden[5] asserts that these postulates have not been completely met. He states, however, that consistent descriptions of *H pylori* are present in duodenal ulcer patients around the world. To better fulfill the postulates, he suggests, it is necessary to prove that infection with *H pylori* precedes development of ulcerative disease. Several prospective studies have addressed that question[8,9] histologically and serologically. We now recognize that *H py-*

lori is typically acquired in childhood and that the clinical manifestations are delayed, often for many decades. Megraud and Lamouliatte point out that Koch himself did not intend for his criteria to be rigidly applied when determining associations between infectious organisms and disease and that the entire concept of chronic disease does not mesh well with the standard use of Koch's postulates.[10]

In 1965, Hill proposed causal criteria to assess an association between lung cancer and smoking.[11] The first criterion is the strength of the association, which is strong for *H pylori* and duodenal ulcer regardless of location, method, or protocol. The second criterion, as applied to *H pylori*, is the temporal relationship between the infection and ulcer development. *H pylori* unambiguously precedes the onset of ulcer disease. Criterion number three relates to the existence of a biologic gradient consistent with causation. This criterion must include acid secretion because acid secretion (or more properly, duodenal acid load) appears to be a biologic gradient that links *H pylori* and duodenal ulcer disease (see below). The fourth criterion addresses how an organism that typically infects the antrum could cause ulcers in the duodenum. Megraud and Lamouliatte emphasize the well-known tendency of *H pylori* to bind to areas of gastric metaplasia in the duodenal bulb such that *H pylori* and gastric metaplasia are constant features of *H pylori*-related duodenal ulcer disease.[10] Hill's fifth criterion links interventions in the disease process and causation of the organism in the disease. This is consistent with cure of the infection eliminating ulcer recurrence. The final criterion addresses the correlation between the understanding of duodenal ulcer disease and the theory that *H pylori* is causative. This criterion is the focus of many investigators studying the effect of *H pylori* infection on gastroduodenal structure and function.

Duodenal Acid Load in Duodenal Disease

The concept of 'no acid, no ulcer' introduced by Schwarz in the last century remains valid. One major focus of research in the pathogenesis of duodenal ulcer has been the search for a dysregulation in acid secretion that would explain the disease. The abnormalities in gastroduodenal physiology include an exaggerated meal-stimulated gastrin release; a larger-than-normal parietal cell mass with concomitant increase in maximum acid output; an upward shift of the dose response of acid secretion to infusion of gastrin-releasing peptide; failure of antral acidification to normally inhibit acid secretion; failure of antral distention to stimulate acid secretion; and an abnormally low duodenal bulb bicarbonate response to instillation of acid. With the exception of increase in parietal cell mass, these phenomena have been shown to be reversible epiphenomena related to *H pylori* infection.[12,13] A unifying hypothesis relates increased duodenal acid load, *H pylori*, and duodenal ulcer disease. The critical factor is that lowering the pH in the duodenum below the pK_a for bile acids would remove the bile acids that normally inhibit growth of *H pylori* (see Chapter 3). The abnormalities in gastroduodenal physiology associated with *H pylori* infection all increase duodenal acid load. Other factors that may also increase the duodenal acid load are smoking and stress (Figure 6). The corollary is that reducing the duodenal acid load with antisecretory drugs or antacids not only would help accelerate ulcer healing, but also would make the environment in the duodenal bulb inhospitable for growth of *H pylori*.

Duodenal Ulcer Disease Protects Against Gastric Cancer

An apparent paradox is that two *H pylori*-associated diseases seem to be mutually exclusive. The presence or history of duodenal ulcer disease protects against development of gastric cancer. The low risk of gastric cancer in patients with duodenal ulcer has been confirmed in recent epidemiologic studies evaluating the risk of *H pylori* infection for the development of gastric carcinoma.

At the beginning of the 20th century, gastric cancer was common and duodenal ulcer rare. During the first

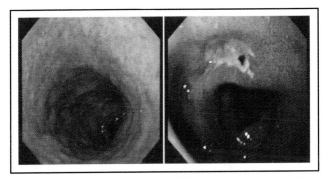

Figure 6: A normal duodenal bulb is contrasted with a duodenal bulb with an active ulcer. The bulb with the ulcer is deformed, scarred, and smaller than the normal bulb. The mucosa is more inflamed, and a greater proportion of the mucosa is not villose but rather gastric metaplasia that has the capacity to secrete acid locally in the bulb. Not surprisingly, the two organs have significant differences in function (eg, bicarbonate response to an acid load). Cure of the infection results in gradual return toward normal.

half of that century, the prevalence of gastric cancer fell while that of duodenal ulcer rose. The development of a new disease (duodenal ulcer) was reminiscent of the other new diseases appearing about the same time, paralytic polio and infectious hepatitis. Both were infectious diseases that were not new but rather had different manifestations in infants and in older individuals. We proposed that the change in the epidemiology of duodenal ulcer/gastric cancer also related to the age at which the patient acquired the infection. In this hypothesis, people who become infected at an early age have many years to develop gastric inflammation, and if the infection occurred in young children, they were likely to progress to atrophic gastritis. The development of atrophic gastritis would in turn diminish acid secretion to below the level required to develop duodenal ulcer disease. In contrast, development of the infection at a later age would allow the gastric corpus to remain relatively spared and promote duodenal ulcer. Many investigators have adopted the 'age of acquisition hypothesis' as true. Unfortunately, the epidemiologic data have not supported the hypothesis. In numerous examples of regions such as Bangladesh where *H pylori* infection is acquired early in childhood, duodenal ulcer disease is common, and gastric cancer is rare.[14] Another example is China, where the age of acquisition in childhood is similar in different regions, yet the prevalence of duodenal ulcer disease and gastric cancer varies remarkably. We now believe that the age of acquisition of atrophic gastritis rather than simply the age of acquisition of the infection is the most important determinant of later development of gastric cancer. The outcome, atrophic pangastritis, is likely a function of three interrelated factors: *H pylori* strains, environment (diet), and host factors.

Epidemiologic research showing significant geographic differences in the prevalence of gastric carcinoma has been more helpful in explaining the pronounced differences in areas with similar *H pylori* prevalence. The incidence of a particular outcome (eg, gastric cancer) can change rapidly over time or with migration despite the fact that neither host genetic makeup nor the predominant strain of *H pylori* in the population has changed. The most likely explanation seems to be crucial environmental differences that allow the combination of host and strain differences to promote early development of atrophic pangastritis. Differences in diet seem most likely, but more research to investigate these possibilities is clearly needed.

Gastric Cancer

The association between gastritis and gastric cancer was recognized decades before the discovery of *H pylori* as a cause of gastritis. The link to *H pylori* infection was confirmed after the discovery of the pathogenic role of the organism in gastritis.[15,16] Although the incidence of gastric adenocarcinoma in the United States has steadily declined for the past 50 years, gastric cancer was the most common cancer in the early part of the 20th century (Figure 7) and remains the second most frequent fatal cancer in the world. Even now, the lifetime risk of developing gastric cancer is 1% to 3% in the United States, and in many countries it remains the first or second most common cancer. For example, in Korea, the likelihood that an adult male will die of gastric cancer is greater than 7%. In 1994, the World Health Organization's (WHO) International Agency for Research on Cancer classified *H pylori* as a definite carcinogen (in the WHO classification system for putative environmental and biologic carcinogens).[17] This classification was largely based on the epidemiologic links and not on a specific pathogenic pathway.

Epidemiologic Links

Gastric cancer is typically separated histologically into two types: an intestinal form strongly related to *H pylori* infection and a diffuse form where the association is positive but weaker. The incidence of gastric cancer usually parallels that of *H pylori* infection in countries with a high incidence of gastric cancer and is consistent with *H pylori* as the cause of the precursor lesion, chronic atrophic gastritis.[18] The strongest epidemiologic evidence for a link between the infection and later development of gastric adenocarcinoma comes from serologic studies demonstrating that people infected with *H pylori* have a higher incidence of gastric carcinoma. Serologic tests are appropriate because antibodies to *H pylori* document even remote exposures, whereas biopsy-based studies of gastric adenocarcinoma may miss prior *H pylori* infection because *H pylori* is unable to colonize adenocarcinoma tissue. Prospective studies have demonstrated a link between *H pylori* and gastric cancer, with the time between diagnosis of the infection and discovery of the cancer ranging from

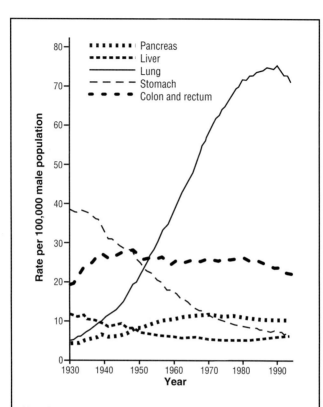

Note: Because of changes in the ICD coding, numerator information has changed over time. Rates for cancer of the liver, lung, and colon and rectum are affected by these coding changes.
Rates are per 100,000 population and are age-adjusted to the 1970 US standard population.
Data source: Vital Statistics of the United States, 1997.

Figure 7: Age-adjusted cancer death rates for males by site, 1930-1994. Used with permission: Landis SH, Murray T, Bolden S, et al: Cancer statistics, 1998. *CA Cancer J Clin* 1998;48:6-29.

6 to 14 years with matched odds ratios from 2.2 to 6.0. In the EUROGAST Study Group, *H pylori* infection increased the risk of gastric cancer by a factor of 6.[19] These odds ratios greatly underestimate the strength of the association. Gastric cancer is a rare disease among populations with a low prevalence of *H pylori* infection. Prior and current histologic studies have repeatedly shown that chronic gastritis was the precursor lesion for gastric cancer. Odds ratios reflect the background prevalence of the factor in the population such that in populations where *H pylori* infection is common, the odds ratios will be low, but the incidence of cancer will be high. To achieve high odds ratios, one must have a low background rate of *H pylori* infection. This can easily be seen by looking at the odds ratios among gastric cancer patients who are young (Figure 8). Few dispute that smoking is related to lung cancer, yet if everyone smoked the odds ratio would be 1. In countries where gastric cancer is common, almost everyone is infected.

The risk of developing gastric cancer can be predicted based on the pattern of histology. For example, among those with antral predominant gastritis and normal to high acid secretion, the risk of duodenal ulcer is in the range of 1% per year, and the risk of gastric cancer approaches 0% per year. The opposite is true for those with atrophic pangastritis, in whom the risk of gastric cancer is approximately 1% per year, and the risk of duodenal ulcer is 0%. There is no question that *H pylori* is etiologically related to both diseases, but one must know more than whether the infection is present to define the risk for a particular patient. A recent follow-up study from Japan illustrates what actually happens. In follow-up of approximately 1 decade, no gastric cancer developed in those without *H pylori*, those whose *H pylori* was cured, or those with antral predominant gastritis. In contrast, those with active *H pylori* and severe atrophic pangastritis had an incidence of new gastric cancer of approximately 1% per year (Figure 9), confirming the association of *H pylori* with gastric cancer and the importance of the histologic pattern and severity of gastritis with outcome. Such studies point out the keys to defining the question regarding the changes that have occurred in *H pylori*-related diseases such as gastric cancer and duodenal ulcer in the 20th century. The question that should be asked is "why did the patterns of gastritis change?" That question allows one to focus on the changes in the environment and diet and thus begin to understand why and how the patterns of disease changed.

As will be examined later, there is no association of *H pylori* infection with adenocarcinoma of the lower esophagus or gastric cardia, which is consistent with those tumors' association with normal or high acid secretion and with Barrett's esophagus and gastroesophageal reflux disease.

Possible Mechanism

There is no single mechanism for development of gastric carcinoma after *H pylori* infection. Cancer is typically multifactorial. Acute gastritis is the initial lesion, progressing in some to multifocal atrophic gastritis. The sequence of events leading to gastric cancer is *H pylori* infection, superficial gastritis, atrophy, development of increasingly severe intestinal metaplasia, dysplasia, and finally invasive carcinoma (Figures 8 and 9).

The role of increased cell turnover or elaboration of toxic oxygen free radicals in the damaging effects of chronic *H pylori* infection is under investigation. However, neither is likely to be critical by itself because both are also present in patients with duodenal ulcer disease.[20] The extent of intestinal metaplasia seems to be a crucial predictor of cancer, but it may simply be a marker for the presence of low acid secretion or the extent of atrophy.[21] We have proposed that once the precursor lesion of chronic atrophic gastritis is present, the risk of developing gastric carcinoma can be calculated per year and per lifetime. This statistical chance is akin to the way we think about the cancer risk associated with sun-induced skin damage, chronic ulcerative colitis, or Barrett's esophagus. The risk

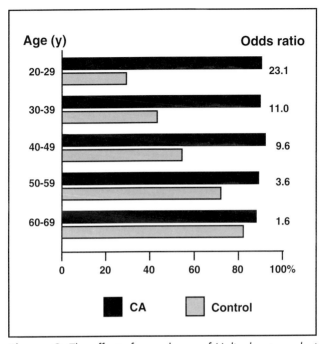

Figure 8: The effect of prevalence of *Helicobacter pylori* on the odds ratio of *H pylori* to gastric cancer. The fall in prevalence of *H pylori* in Japan has been associated with a fall in the prevalence of gastric cancer. In young individuals, *H pylori* infection is uncommon and increases with age. In contrast, the proportion of gastric cancer patients with *H pylori* infection is high in every age group. This figure illustrates the critical effect of prevalence of *H pylori* in the population on the resulting odds ratio such that while the biology does not change (most gastric cancers are caused by *H pylori*), the odds ratio is greatly influenced. Adapted from Kituchi S, Wada O, Nakajima T, et al: Association between gastric cancer and *H pylori* with reference to age. *Gut* 1995;37(suppl 1):A8.

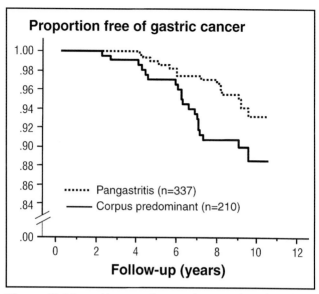

Figure 9: Natural history of a population with *Helicobacter pylori*-related protection against gastroesophageal reflux disease (GERD). Kaplan-Meier analysis of the proportion of patients with *H pylori* related to pangastritis or corpus predominant gastritis who remained free of gastric cancer. This illustrates that the histologic patterns of gastritis that are characteristic of 'protection' against GERD are those most likely associated with gastric cancer. Adapted from Uemura N, Okumoto S, Yamamoto S, et el: *Helicobacter pylori* infection and the development of gastric cancer. *N Engl J Med* 2001;345:784-789.

for the population is calculated as the risk per year times the number of years of exposure. The risk to the population can be increased by behavior that promotes cancer (eg, cigarette smoking, high-salt diet) or decreased by the consumption of fresh fruits and vegetables.[22] The highest rates of gastric carcinoma are found in populations that have an accelerated acquisition of chronic atrophic gastritis. Infection early in life maximizes the risk. Using the calculation of risk times years of exposure, gastric cancer rates are expected to be low in countries where the rate of developing atrophic gastritis is low, even if *H pylori* infection is prevalent.

Molecular Mimicry as Basis for Gastric Atrophy

Although chronic inflammation is a sufficient cause for progressive damage and loss of cellular elements, other explanations also are possible, including one based on molecular mimicry.[23,24] A study of 100 patients with positive *H pylori* serologic tests found that most had autoantibodies that cross-reacted with gastric antigens. The autoantibody activity was primarily along the gastric glandular epithelium, especially the cytoplasmic apical border of chief and parietal cells. The autoantibody reaction was most pronounced at the neck region of the gland, decreasing toward the glandular bases, with a striking correlation between lymphocytic involvement in the neck epithelial cells and the presence of autoantibodies. Researchers have suggested that the antibodies may be formed in a cross-reaction against cryptic mucin epitopes that were exposed during regeneration of the gastric epithelium. Patients with autoantibodies had a much higher frequency of glandular atrophy and lymphocytic infiltration than did autoantibody-negative *H pylori* patients, suggesting that a chronic autoimmune attack against the gastric epithelium may be involved in the progression of gastritis to atrophy with metaplastic changes.

The molecular mimicry involved mucin glycoproteins, and studies have shown that *H pylori* expresses O-side chain polysaccharides with blood group determinants, including Le^x and Le^y.[25] These same antigens are present in normal glandular gastric epithelium, suggesting that the molecular mimicry may be based on blood group antigenic determinants. Patients with the most au-

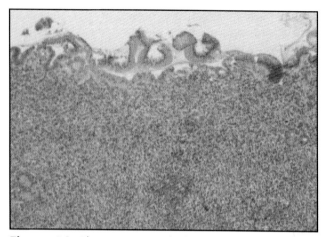

Figure 10: Photomicrograph showing extensive infiltration of the gastric mucosa with a monoclonal population of B lymphocytes associated with destruction and invasion of normal glandular elements.

toantibodies also had more severe pathologic findings such that the grade of antigenic mimicry appeared to correlate with the tendency to develop atrophy. Because the prevalence of gastritis with atrophy varies geographically and regionally, it seems unlikely that the presence of molecular mimicry can explain the entire picture. More studies are needed.

Primary Gastric B-Cell Lymphoma (MALT Lymphoma)

The normal stomach lacks organized lymphoid tissue, but after infection with *H pylori*, lymphoid tissue is universally present. Acquisition of gastric lymphoid tissue is believed to be caused by persistent antigen stimulation from by-products of chronic *H pylori* infection.[26] After the lymphoid tissue is stimulated into forming MALT, genetic damage in these cells can occur over time, leading to development of gastric lymphoma. MALT lymphomas are monoclonal proliferations of cancerous B cells that have infiltrated gastric glands (Figure 10). Gastric MALT lymphomas are typically low-grade T-cell-dependent B-cell lymphomas whose antigenic stimulus is believed to be *H pylori*. The association between gastric MALT lymphoma and chronic gastritis preceded the discovery of *H pylori*, and the association has recently been confirmed by demonstration of strong epidemiologic associations between *H pylori* and gastric MALT lymphoma.[27,28]

Can Cancer Be Cured by Eradication of *Helicobacter pylori* Infection?

Gastric adenocarcinoma cannot be cured by eradication of *H pylori* infection. Gastric cancer can theoretically be prevented by prevention of atrophic gastritis. Because the risk of developing gastric cancer is significantly increased in first-degree relatives of patients with gastric cancer, these relatives should probably be tested for the presence of the infection, and those who prove to be infected should be treated. Whether cure of the infection reverses severe dysplasia (eg, carcinoma in situ) is controversial. In our limited experience, it does not. Nevertheless, data from Japan suggest that cure of the infection after treatment of the primary gastric cancer is associated with a reduced rate of development of new primary cancer.[29] Because there is no reason not to treat the *H pylori* infection after curative cancer therapy, treatment of *H pylori* is recommended.

In contrast to the dismal results with gastric adenocarcinoma, cure of *H pylori* infection results in remission of MALT lymphoma in most cases. Complete resolution may take 6 to 12 months, and the lymphoma may recur with the reacquisition of *H pylori* infection. The general approach to the presence of low-grade gastric MALT lymphoma is to: (1) confirm that it is localized to the stomach, (2) cure the *H pylori* infection, and (3) follow the course of the disease endoscopically and clinically. Importantly, the diagnosis of MALT lymphoma is often made incidentally during a work-up for some separate condition. In our experience, MALT lymphomas usually present as grossly normal-appearing mucosa, but on histologic examination the neoplastic B-cell population is found to exhibit typical MALT lymphoma morphology. Monoclonality is confirmed by genetic testing of the biopsies.

Other Gastrointestinal Associations

Nonulcer Dyspepsia

Dyspepsia has numerous causes, including gastroesophageal reflux disease, peptic ulcer disease, and drug use (eg, NSAIDs), and can be idiopathic. The concept of nonulcer dyspepsia implies that the patient has undergone investigations to confirm the absence of ulcer disease; therefore, it might be better called *investigated dyspepsia*. The population presenting with *uninvestigated dyspepsia* will have a higher proportion of patients with *H pylori* peptic ulcer. As will be examined later, the recommended approach for such patients is to assess for alarm symptoms or red flags that would prompt endoscopy and, if absent, test for *H pylori*. Those who are infected with *H pylori* receive therapy. Although some cases of investigated nonulcer dyspepsia undoubtedly are linked to *H pylori* infection, it is impossible to identify these cases because the frequency of *H pylori* in patients with nonulcer dyspepsia is roughly equal to that in patients who are asymptomatic. Also, prospective trials of antimicrobial therapy directed against *H pylori* in nonulcer dyspepsia patients have been somewhat disappointing.[30,31] Meta-analyses have shown that approximately 10% of patients will have sustained remission (cure) of their symptoms. Even though symptoms may remain, curing the infection will likely prevent subsequent development of peptic ulcer, should markedly reduce or prevent development of gastric cancer, and will eliminate the individual from the reservoir of infected individuals responsible for the maintenance of the infection within the population.[32,33]

NSAID-Induced Ulcer Disease

NSAIDs are used daily by millions of Americans, a significant number of whom develop ulcerative complications. Some studies suggest NSAID use is the most important risk factor for developing complicated ulcer disease.[34] Because *H pylori* is present in most duodenal and gastric ulcer patients, the interaction between *H pylori* and NSAID use is of great interest.

A number of prospective studies looked at gastric injury and frank ulcer formation in *H pylori*-positive patients before and after ingesting NSAIDs.[34] A recent study reported a correlation between the presence of *H pylori* and risk of ulcer development in patients taking NSAIDs who did not have ulcers at the beginning of the study.[35] This was a prospective study in Hong Kong. Patients with *H pylori* infection but no preexisting ulcers on endoscopy were randomly assigned naproxen alone (750 mg daily) for 8 weeks or a 1-week course of triple therapy (bismuth subcitrate 120 mg, tetracycline 500 mg, and metronidazole [Flagyl®, Protostat®] 400 mg, each given orally four times daily) before naproxen administration. Endoscopy was repeated after 8 weeks of naproxen treatment or when naproxen treatment was stopped early because of bleeding or intractable dyspepsia. Twelve patients (26%) with persistent *H pylori* infection and one (3%) with successful *H pylori* therapy developed ulcers with naproxen (P=0.002). The results of this study are provocative and suggest that patients receiving long-term NSAID therapy should be tested for *H pylori*. Several caveats apply. First, a 26% ulcer incidence in 8 weeks exceeds expectations based on the large number of clinical trials. In our study, we separated those with *H pylori* infection from those without to examine the risk of developing ulcers for arthritic patients taking NSAIDs. We did not find an increased risk in those with *H pylori* infection.[36] A study from Italy also examined recurrent ulcers in those whose *H pylori* infection was cured and found no statistical difference.[37] Thus, we believe it is best to be aware of the results of the study from Hong Kong but not to implement a test-and-treat strategy until more information is available.

Researchers have proposed that *H pylori* infection with concomitant NSAID use may additively increase the risk of bleeding.[38] The highest probability of bleeding has been in *H pylori*-positive patients who used NSAIDs.[39] Cure of *H pylori* infection should reduce the overall incidence of ulcer disease, although cure of the infection does not eliminate the risk of bleeding in patients who continue to use NSAIDs.[40]

The data regarding an *H pylori*/NSAID interaction are now sufficiently strong that the recent Maastricht Consensus report suggested that all patients for whom long-term NSAID use is contemplated be tested for *H pylori* and, if the infection is present, receive therapy.[41]

Tenuous Associations

Cure of a Disease With Cure of *Helicobacter pylori* Infection

Treatment with antibiotics may have many effects, including a beneficial effect on infections other than *H pylori* (eg, periodontal disease). Studies are beginning to claim that *H pylori* infection is related to many extragastric conditions, such as headache and diabetes. The association is based on a serologic survey (eg, diabetes) or response to therapy (eg, headache). Response to therapy is a weak argument because placebo response must be considered, as well as response to the antibiotic regimen or other infections (eg, chronic sinusitis). Appropriate controls must include matched individuals with the condition (eg, headache) and without *H pylori* infection, and must demonstrate that cure of the disease is predominantly present in those with *H pylori* infection. The current flurry of reports is reminiscent of the time when all of an individual's teeth were removed in an attempt to eliminate a source of chronic inflammation that was the 'cause' of the disease in question.[42]

Coronary Artery Disease

A number of reports purport to show a relationship between *H pylori* and coronary artery disease. The association is controversial and unlikely, with many conflicting studies and most reports still being presented as letters or abstracts. Mendall et al[43] suggested an increased risk of coronary artery disease associated with *H pylori* infection. Alterations in coagulation studies in *H pylori*-infected patients, including raised fibrinogen levels and increased procoagulant activity from mononuclear cells, have been reported and believed to possibly contribute to ischemic heart disease.[44] However, many studies have opposed the link between *H pylori* and heart disease, suggesting that both are markers of childhood poverty but are not otherwise directly related. For example, Sandifer et al found a negative association between *H pylori* infection and the presence of ischemic heart disease in the EUROGAST Study Group data,[45] as did most recent papers. We conclude that little evidence associates *H pylori* infection and heart disease.

Rosacea

A few case reports have documented resolution of a chronic skin condition, acne rosacea, on treatment of co-existing *H pylori* infections. However, infections respond to antibiotics, and this is equally true of those with rosacea without *H pylori* as it is in those with the infection. This observation is likely another excellent example of poorly controlled observations.

Pernicious Anemia

Pernicious anemia may arise from two mechanisms: a genetic autosomal dominant disease and long-standing *H pylori* infection. Recent data suggest that both pathways lead to vitamin B_{12} malabsorption via absence of intrinsic factor.[46] Thus, *H pylori* and an autoimmune mechanism may lead to pernicious anemia. *H pylori* even can possibly be the trigger for the autoimmune form of the disease. *H pylori*-related pernicious anemia is associated with atrophy of the antrum and the corpus, whereas true autoimmune pernicious anemia has only corpus atrophy.

References

1. Breuer T, Malaty HM, Graham DY: The epidemiology of *H pylori*-associated gastroduodenal diseases. In: Ernst PB, Michetti P, Smith PD, eds. *The Immunobiology of H pylori: From Pathogenesis to Prevention.* Philadelphia, Lippincott-Raven, 1997, pp 1-14.

2. Dixon MF: *Helicobacter pylori* and peptic ulceration: histopathological aspects. *J Gastroenterol Hepatol* 1991;6:125-130.

3. Ota H, Genta RM: Morphological characterization of the gastric mucosa during infection with *H pylori*. In: Ernst PB, Michetti P, Smith PD, eds. *The Immunobiology of H pylori: From Pathogenesis to Prevention.* Philadelphia, Lippincott-Raven, 1997, pp 15-28.

4. Valle J, Kekki M, Sipponen P, et al: Long-term course and consequences of *Helicobacter pylori* gastritis. Results of a 32-year follow-up study. *Scand J Gastroenterol* 1996;31:546-550.

5. Howden CW: Clinical expressions of *Helicobacter pylori* infection. *Am J Med* 1996;100:27S-32S.

6. Graham DY, Genta RM, Go MF, et al: Which is the most important factor in duodenal ulcer pathogenesis: the strain of *Helicobacter pylori* or the host? In: Hunt RH, Tytgat GN, eds. *Helicobacter pylori: Basic Mechanisms to Clinical Cure.* Lancaster, Kluwer Academic Publishers, 1996, pp 85-91.

7. Peura DA: *Helicobacter pylori* and ulcerogenesis. *Am J Med* 1996;100:19S-25S.

8. Sipponen P, Varis K, Fraki O, et al: Cumulative 10-year risk of symptomatic duodenal and gastric ulcer in patients with or without chronic gastritis. A clinical follow-up study of 454 outpatients. *Scand J Gastroenterol* 1990;25:966-973.

9. Blaser MJ, Chyou PH, Nomura A: Age at establishment of *Helicobacter pylori* infection and gastric carcinoma, gastric ulcer, and duodenal ulcer risk. *Cancer Res* 1995;55:562-565.

10. Megraud F, Lamouliatte H: *Helicobacter pylori* and duodenal ulcer. Evidence suggesting causation. *Dig Dis Sci* 1992;37:769-772.

11. Hill AB, Hill ID: *Bradford Hill's Principles of Medical Statistics*, 12th ed. London, Edward Arnold, 1991.

12.   Graham DY, Dore MP: Perturbations in gastric physiology in *Helicobacter pylori* duodenal ulcer disease: are they all epiphenomena? *Helicobacter* 1997;2:S44-S49.

13.   Graham DY: *Helicobacter pylori* and perturbations in acid secretion: the end of the beginning. *Gastroenterology* 1996;110:1647-1650.

14.   Graham DY: *Helicobacter pylori* infection in the pathogenesis of duodenal ulcer and gastric cancer: a model. *Gastroenterology* 1997;113:1983-1991.

15.   Asaka M, Sepulveda AR, Sugiyama T, et al: Gastric cancer. In: Mobley HL, Mendz GL, Hazell SL, eds. *Helicobacter pylori: Physiology and Genetics*. Washington, DC, ASM Press, 2001, pp 481-498.

16.   Graham DY: *Helicobacter pylori* infection is the primary cause of gastric cancer. *J Gastroenterol* 2000;35(suppl 12):90-97.

17.   IARC Monographs on the Evaluation of Carcinogenic Risks to Humans: *Schistosomes, Liver Flukes and* Helicobacter pylori, vol. 61. Lyon, France, International Agency for Research on Cancer, 1994.

18.   Correa P: *Helicobacter pylori* and gastric cancer: state of the art. *Cancer Epidemiol Biomarkers Prev* 1996;5:477-481.

19.   An international association between *Helicobacter pylori* infection and gastric cancer. The EUROGAST Study Group. *Lancet* 1993;341:1359-1362.

20.   Graham DY, Go MF, Genta RM: *Helicobacter pylori*, duodenal ulcer, gastric cancer: tunnel vision or blinders? *Ann Med* 1995;27:589-594.

21.   Lechago J, Correa P: Prolonged achlorhydria and gastric neoplasia: is there a causal relationship? *Gastroenterology* 1993; 104:1554-1557.

22.   Hwang H, Dwyer J, Russell RM: Diet, *Helicobacter pylori* infection, food preservation and gastric cancer risk: are there new roles for preventative factors? *Nutr Rev* 1994;52:75-83.

23.   Appelmelk BJ, Negrini R, Moran AP, et al: Molecular mimicry between *Helicobacter pylori* and the host. *Trends Microbiol* 1997;5:70-73.

24.   Negrini R, Savio A, Poiesi C, et al: Antigenic mimicry between *Helicobacter pylori* and gastric mucosa in the pathogenesis of body atrophic gastritis. *Gastroenterology* 1996;111:655-665.

25.   Appelmelk BJ, Simoons-Smit I, Negrini R, et al: Potential role of molecular mimicry between *Helicobacter pylori* lipopolysac-

charide and host Lewis blood group antigens in autoimmunity. *Infect Immun* 1996;64:2031-2040.

26. Sorrentino D, Ferraccioli GF, DeVita S, et al: B-cell clonality and infection with *Helicobacter pylori*: implications for development of gastric lymphoma. *Gut* 1996;38:837-840.

27. Parsonnet J, Hansen S, Rodriguez L, et al: *Helicobacter pylori* infection and gastric lymphoma. *N Engl J Med* 1994;330:1267-1271.

28. Carlson SJ, Yokoo H, Vanagunas A: Progression of gastritis to monoclonal B-cell lymphoma with resolution and recurrence following eradication of *Helicobacter pylori*. *JAMA* 1996;275:937-939.

29. Uemura N, Mukai T, Okamato S, et al: Effect of *Helicobacter pylori* eradication on subsequent development of cancer after endoscopic resection of early gastric cancer. *Cancer Epidemiol Biomarkers Prev* 1997;6:639-642.

30. Talley NJ: *Helicobacter pylori* and non-ulcer dyspepsia. *Scand J Gastroenterol Suppl* 1996;220:19-22.

31. Talley NJ: A critique of therapeutic trials in *Helicobacter pylori*-positive functional dyspepsia. *Gastroenterology* 1994;106:1174-1183.

32. Moayyedi P, Soo S, Deeks J, et al: Eradication of *Helicobacter pylori* for non-ulcer dyspepsia. *Cochrane Database Syst Rev* 2001;CD002096.

33. Moayyedi P, Soo S, Deeks J, et al: Systematic review and economic evaluation of *Helicobacter pylori* eradication treatment for non-ulcer dyspepsia. Dyspepsia Review Group. *BMJ* 2000; 321:659-664.

34. Laine LA: *Helicobacter pylori* and complicated ulcer disease. *Am J Med* 1996;100:52S-59S.

35. Chan FK, Sung JJ, Chung SC, et al: Randomised trial of eradication of *Helicobacter pylori* before non-steroidal anti-inflammatory drug therapy to prevent peptic ulcers. *Lancet* 1997;350:975-979.

36. Kim JG, Graham DY: *Helicobacter pylori* infection and development of gastric or duodenal ulcer in arthritic patients receiving chronic NSAID therapy. The Misoprostol Study Group. *Am J Gastroenterol* 1994;89:203-207.

37. Bianchi Porro G, Parente F, Imbesi V, et al: Role of *Helicobacter pylori* in ulcer healing and recurrence of gastric and duodenal ulcers in longterm NSAID users. Response to omeprazole dual therapy. *Gut* 1996;39:22-26.

38. Graham DY: Nonsteroidal anti-inflammatory drugs, *Helicobacter pylori*, and ulcers: where we stand. *Am J Gastroenterol* 1996;91:2080-2086.

39. al-Assi MT, Genta RM, Karttunen TJ, et al: Ulcer site and complications: relation to *Helicobacter pylori* infection and NSAID use. *Endoscopy* 1996;28:229-233.

40. Bazzoli F, De Luca L, Graham DY: *Helicobacter pylori* infection and the use of NSAIDs. *Best Pract Res Clin Gastroenterol* 2001;15:775-778.

41. Malfertheiner P, Megraud F, O'Morain C, et al: Current concepts in the management of *Helicobacter pylori* infection—the Maastricht 2-2000 consensus report. *Aliment Pharmacol Ther* 2002;16:167-180.

42. Davis A: The emergence of American dental medicine: the relation of the maxillary antrum to focal infection. *Tex Rep Biol Med* 1974;32:141-156.

43. Mendall MA, Goggin PM, Molineaux N, et al: Relation of *Helicobacter pylori* infection and coronary heart disease. *Br Heart J* 1994;71:437-439.

44. Patel P, Carrington D, Strachan DP, et al: Fibrinogen: a link between chronic infection and coronary heart disease. *Lancet* 1994;343:1634-1635.

45. Sandifer QD, Vuilo S, Crompton G: Association of *Helicobacter pylori* infection with coronary heart disease. Association may not be causal. *BMJ* 1996;312:251.

46. Annibale B, Marignani M, Azzoni C, et al: Atrophic body gastritis: distinct features associated with *Helicobacter pylori* infection. *Helicobacter* 1997;2:57-64.

Chapter 5

Diagnostic Tests

T he clear links between *Helicobacter pylori* and a number of important gastrointestinal diseases prompted development of a variety of methods to detect the presence of the infection. Diagnostic tests for *H pylori* can be broadly classified into two categories: invasive tests that require endoscopy and noninvasive or minimally invasive tests that do not. This chapter also addresses the clinical settings in which each test is most appropriate and who, in general, should undergo testing for *H pylori* infection.

Invasive Tests

The gold standard for the presence of most infectious diseases is successful culture of the organism. *H pylori* is easily grown in the laboratory, but a high rate of success depends on experience. The organism is fastidious in its growth requirements and in the requirements for transport from the endoscopy suite to the laboratory.[1] Transport from the endoscopy suite may require changing normal routines with formalin-fixed specimens because delay in reaching the laboratory, drying of the biopsy sample, and poor choice of transport medium all reduce the successful culture rate.[2] The typical laboratory reports success rates in culturing the organism between 70% and 80%, with a 90% to 95% sensitivity and 100% specificity. Experienced laboratories in research units do better. Ideally, gastric mucosal biopsies should immediately be placed in transport media and taken to the laboratory. If processing will occur within 2 hours, saline can be used as the transport medium. Otherwise, specimens should be transported in a glycerol-containing medium. In an emergency, samples may be stored in a glycerol-containing medium such as skim milk/glycerol, brucella broth/glycerol, or cysteine-Albimi/glycerol at 4°C for up to 1 week but with some loss of recoverability.[2] Biopsies can be safely stored without loss of *H pylori* recoverability at -20°C for 4 weeks and indefinitely at -70°C. At room temperature after 6 hours, the *H pylori* titer is reduced, and by 48 hours most cultures will be negative.

Because antibiotic resistance is becoming widespread among *H pylori*, pretreatment culture will become increasingly important. Unless new antibiotic regimens are developed, determination of susceptibility patterns may soon be required before choosing the appropriate therapy.

Histology as a Gold Standard

Normal gastric mucosa is devoid of inflammatory cells. Because *H pylori* infection is associated with marked infiltration of the mucosa with acute and chronic inflammatory cells, histology potentially has many advantages for detection of the presence of the infection. In fact, the current gold standard for detection of *H pylori* is histologic examination of endoscopic mucosal biopsy specimens using a special stain.[3,4] Hematoxylin-eosin (H&E) stain alone has proven unsatisfactory because of lack of sufficient sensitivity for detection of the organism. Warthin-Starry silver-based staining has had success, but it has the problems of high background, fading over time, expense, and lack of optimal preservation of tissue architecture.[3] Giemsa and Diff-Quik® staining also have proved useful. Unfortunately, none of these special stains allows for adequate visualization of the gastric morphology. Thus, two stains are required (eg, H&E plus a special stain). Triple stains that combine H&E, Alcian blue, and another stain to identify the bacterium such as the Genta or El-Zimaity triple stains allow easy identification of *H pylori* and excellent visualization of gastric morphology (Figure 1). The original Genta stain used uranyl nitrate, which is not avail-

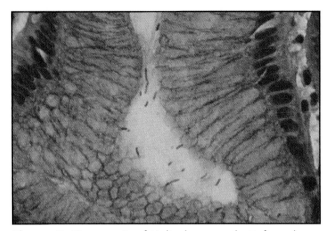

Figure 1: Genta stain of *Helicobacter pylori*-infected gastric mucosa showing not only the inflammatory infiltration, but also numerous bacteria on the mucosal surface.

able widely, and the staining technique was not suitable for use with an autostainer. Recent modifications include replacing uranyl nitrate with a lead nitrate-gum mastic solution and using a microwave oven for the sensitization, silver impregnation, and reduction steps. This reduced the staining time to 28 minutes. The technical time can be reduced to 9 to 10 minutes if deparaffinization and all steps following reduction are done with the help of an autostainer.[5]

Our laboratory routinely uses the Genta (Figure 1) or El-Zimaity triple stains, which require only one slide. For those laboratories that use a special stain only when there is a possibility of *H pylori* (eg, when the mucosa shows inflammation) and post-therapy, we recommend the use of the Diff-Quik® stain because it is readily available, rapid, and inexpensive.[6] When only a few bacteria are present and there is a question about whether a case is positive or negative, we use the El-Zimaity dual stain, which combines periodic acid Schiff (PAS) and a silver stain.[7]

> ## Table 1: Recommendations for Collecting Gastric Mucosal Biopsies for Detection of *Helicobacter pylori*
>
> - Use jumbo or large-cup forceps
> - Biopsy normal-appearing mucosa
> - Take multiple (at least four) biopsies: two antral and two corpus
> - Do not handle or orient specimens; rather, 'shake off' into formalin
> - Encourage pathologist to use a special stain and to report results using the New Sydney system[9]

This is also the only practical way to visualize *H pylori* in the duodenal mucosa.

Failure to include a special stain may cause a false-negative result in up to 25%, especially in post-treatment patients. Immunohistochemistry is used in some laboratories but is inferior to the triple stains or the dual stain for *H pylori* diagnosis.

Histology also provides a permanent record and thus should be the ideal method of diagnosis. Despite the success with histology, many practical limitations have made the results less than ideal. The problems relate to the location, number, handling, and processing of the tissue specimens; the skill of the histologic technician in embedding and staining; and the ability and interest of the histopathologist reviewing the biopsy material. Thus, potential problems occur at many steps in the process, from collection of the specimens to their interpretation.[8]

H pylori is located superficially in the mucus layer and attached to the surface. This superficial location requires that the specimens not be damaged during handling and that they be embedded correctly (Table 1). The patholo-

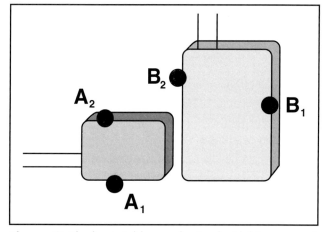

Figure 2: The best yields are obtained with biopsy specimen obtained from predetermined locations. We recommend one from the lesser curvature and one from the greater curvature of the corpus and the antrum. We prefer to place the corpus and antral specimens into separate bottles. A = antrum, B = body or corpus.

gist can review only whatever specimens are submitted. The larger the specimen, the more likely the histologic technician and the pathologist will be able to practice their crafts well. Using large-cup biopsy forceps (eg, Micro-Vasive®, Radial Jaw™) and taking biopsies from the antrum and corpus will provide a good yield. Because the organisms may be distributed unequally around the stomach and are absent or difficult to visualize in areas of intestinal metaplasia, biopsies from the lesser and greater curvature are recommended. Two antral biopsies, including one from the gastric angle, and two corpus biopsies are preferred[9] (Figure 2). To prevent removal of the gastric mucus, no attempt should be made to orient the biopsies before fixation. Rather, the histology technician must

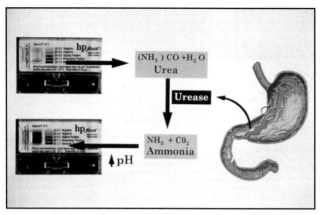

Figure 3: *Helicobacter pylori* urease liberates ammonia from urease in the medium. The resulting increase in pH is observed as a change in the color of a pH indicator dye.

be trained to embed the specimens on edge to ensure that the surface of the mucosa can be visualized. Many pathologists still deny the need to always use a special stain and, in our experience, this results in a false-negative rate of at least 25%, especially post-therapy (ie, the gold standard is sometimes brass). The clinician can obtain a reasonable idea of the accuracy of the pathologist by comparing the results of the pathology with rapid urease testing.

Rapid Urease Tests

Rapid urease tests (RUTs) are based on the fact that *H pylori* contains a large amount of urease enzyme, which splits urea into ammonia and CO_2. When an *H pylori*-containing gastric biopsy is placed into a urea-containing medium, the ammonia produced by *H pylori* urease will increase the pH, which is easily detected by the color change of a pH indicator (Figure 3). Three tests are commercially available in the United States (Figure 4), but any laboratory can easily produce a successful medium. The formula

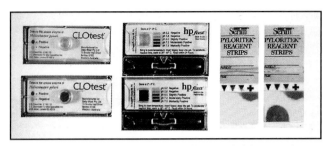

Figure 4: The three commercially available rapid urease tests available in the United States.

for a homemade test is to make a solution containing 2 g urea, 10 mL of 0.5% (weight/volume) phenol red, and 20 mg sodium azide in 100 mL of 0.01 mol/L sodium phosphate buffer, pH 6.5. A 0.5 mL dram vial is filled with 50 µL of this solution, and biopsy specimens are added in the endoscopy room. The test is positive if the medium changes from orange to definite pink. Two of the commercial tests use urea-impregnated agar (*hp*fast, GI Supply; and CLOtest®, TriMed Specialties, Inc.). Another test uses a urea-impregnated semipermeable membrane for ammonia gas (PyloriTek®, Serim). The sensitivity and specificity for these RUTs is between 90% and 95%. The speed of the reaction in the agar tests can be increased by using a warmer (eg, Helicoview, GI Supply), using large biopsy specimens, or adding several specimens to the agar. The PyloriTek® test can be read after 1 hour. The *hp*fast has the theoretic advantages of containing a cell wall detergent and a lower starting pH to take advantage of the fact that *H pylori* urease has a low pH optimum, whereas other potential microbial contaminants do not. There is little practical difference among the available tests; all are inexpensive and can be done easily and rapidly in the endoscopy suite.

The high sensitivities and specificities of RUTs have led many physicians to consider a positive RUT the only required diagnostic test. One cost-saving method uses a tiered approach to diagnostic testing, attempting to reduce costs by eliminating the high cost of processing mucosal biopsies for histology. Biopsies for histology are taken but are retained in the endoscopy suite until the results of the RUT are known. If the RUT is positive, the other biopsy specimens are discarded; if the RUT is negative, these samples are submitted for histologic examination. Biopsy specimens for RUT or histology are best if taken from normal-appearing mucosa, and it is probably safe to discard them. Specimens taken from abnormal-appearing mucosa, or from ulcer margins, should not be used for RUT and should be submitted for histologic evaluation.

RUTs require a high density of bacteria, and anything that reduces the bacterial load may produce false-negative tests. Common events that may transiently reduce the bacterial load include recent use of antibiotics or bismuth-containing compounds and the use of proton pump inhibitors (PPIs). Because RUTs can miss a low-level infection with *H pylori*, a negative test should not be the sole criterion for absence or cure of *H pylori* infection.

Noninvasive Tests

A number of noninvasive tests have been developed to detect the presence of *H pylori* infection. The least expensive, most widely available, and most convenient are based on detection of a humoral immune response (eg, serologically based techniques). Standard laboratory tests and office-based rapid blood tests are now available.

Serologic Testing

Detection of serum IgG against *H pylori* provides a reliable assessment of current or prior *H pylori* infection. Because the infection is often lifelong, a positive test generally denotes an active infection. Because the antibody test remains positive long after successful treatment of the infection, a positive test result cannot ascertain whether the patient has been adequately treated.

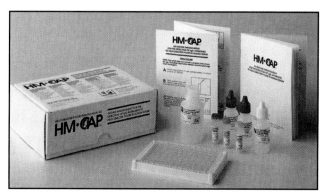

Figure 5: An FDA-approved laboratory test for anti-*Helicobacter pylori* IgG. Results are generally available within 24 hours.

Laboratory-based IgG tests typically use multiwell enzyme-linked immunosorbent assays (ELISA) and are highly sensitive and specific, approaching 95% (Figure 5). The ELISA tests we have evaluated include HM•CAP™ and PyloriStat; both provided excellent results. Some commercial testing laboratories still offer 'in-house'-developed, non-FDA approved tests with unknown (and often poor) sensitivity and specificity (see below).

A number of rapid office-based IgG kits use serum, including QuickVue® (Quidel, San Diego, CA) and FlexSure® *HP* (SmithKline Diagnostics, Palo Alto, CA). Rapid whole-blood-based IgG tests also have become available, but their increased convenience is offset somewhat because the sensitivity and specificities may be slightly lower than serum IgG-based methods (Figure 6).

Test for IgA and IgM Antibodies

Although tests for IgA and IgM to *H pylori* are widely available from commercial sources, only two IgA tests are FDA approved. In our experience, the unapproved tests yield poor and unreliable results and should be

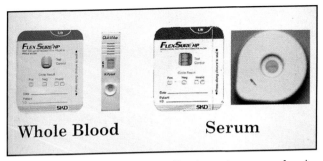

Figure 6: Four rapid, 'in the office' serologic tests for determining the presence of anti-*Helicobacter pylori* IgG. These tests have good specificity and sensitivity. However, because of the slow fall in antibody titers, serologic tests cannot confirm that therapy has been successful.

avoided. Indeed, none of these tests should be used to make therapeutic decisions. In the United States, these tests are labeled *for research only*, and this alone should alert the physician that the test is not FDA approved. In Europe, tests that detect IgM (and IgG) are commercially available (eg, the Malakit *Helicobacter pylori* series from Biolab, Belgium). A Belgian study of 452 asymptomatic children admitted for elective surgery confirmed that the IgA and IgM tests had low sensitivities and specificities and correlated poorly with *H pylori* infection.[10] If the laboratory provides IgM or IgA results, it is using unapproved and inaccurate tests, and a different laboratory should be used.

Saliva and Urine Tests

An attempt has been made to provide diagnostic testing that does not require blood sampling. The first salivary test was the Helisal Assay test (Cortecs Diagnostics, UK), but it has proven to have poor sensitivity and specificity.[11] No salivary test has proven to be reliable, but new tests are in development. Urine tests using immuno-

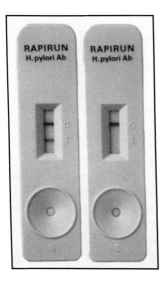

Figure 7: Rapid detection kit for antibodies against *Helicobacter pylori* in urine. The sample is positive when two red bands at the test line and control line are observed 20 minutes later and negative when only the control line is observed.

chromatography have recently become available, including rapid tests. We evaluated the rapid urine test using a test kit (RAPIRUN® *H pylori* Antibody) (Figure 7). We tested 104 individuals, including 43 with *H pylori* infection confirmed by repeatedly positive urea breath tests (UBTs) and 61 *H pylori* negative with repeatedly negative UBTs.[12] Forty-one of the 43 individuals with *H pylori* infection had a positive rapid urine test, with two false-negative tests. There were two false-positive tests among the 61 with repeatedly negative UBTs. The sensitivity, specificity, and positive and negative predictive values for the rapid urine test were 95.3%, 96.7%, 95.3%, and 96.7%, respectively. The kit was easy to use and required no special equipment. The urine tests offer an alternative to serum or whole blood testing but no advantage.

Limitations of Serologic Methods

The chief limitation of serologically based methods is the inability to distinguish active infection from past infection. This becomes a concern in patients who have been previously treated with antibiotics, especially those treated specifically for *H pylori*. Although some researchers have suggested that quantitative serologic testing may be useful in documenting clearance of an infection, this method is reliable only for population surveys and not for individual patients. Even with the availability of paired pre- and post-therapy sera, the specificity and sensitivity of quantitative serologic testing has been poor and should be abandoned as impractical. In addition, as stated in the chapter on epidemiology, in developed countries the prevalence of *H pylori* is declining in every birth cohort tested. Thus, the population of individuals with antibody to *H pylori* but with no infection is increasing. Interpretation of serology results requires an assessment of the pretest probability (eg, likelihood that the patient has or does not have the disease in question). The positive predictive value of the test will depend on the proportion of patients in the population with *H pylori* infection (Figure 8). For example, Figure 8 shows the predictive values for a positive or a negative test with a test with a sensitivity and specificity of 85%. When the prevalence of the disease is less than 30%, a large proportion of tests will be false-positive, but there are essentially no false-negative tests. The opposite occurs when the infection is present in most of the population. Thus, a positive test in a patient with a low likelihood of the infection (eg, a young white American with gastroesophageal reflux disease) would need to be confirmed with a specific test before embarking on anti-*H pylori* therapy. Similarly, a negative serologic test in a patient with a chronic duodenal ulcer disease (high pretest probability) requires confirmation. Most of the available in-the-office or near-patient serologic tests have sensitivities and specificities less than 90% such that unless there is a high pretest probability (a patient with chronic duodenal ulcer disease), most should be confirmed.

The preferred and the best noninvasive test is the nonradioactive ^{13}C UBT, which provides reliable information

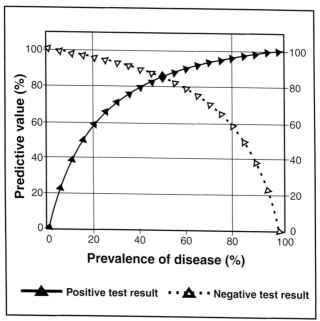

Figure 8: Effect of frequency of *Helicobacter pylori* in a population on the predictive value of a positive or negative test. The effect is shown for tests with specificity and sensitivity (both) of 85%. Low prevalence of *H pylori* results in an increasing proportion of false-positive tests with high accuracy of negative tests. In contrast, when the prevalence of *H pylori* is expected to be high (eg, in duodenal ulcer), false-negative tests become more prevalent. Even at low or high prevalence of *H pylori* infection, the tests retain their stated specificity and sensitivity.

about whether an active *H pylori* infection is present.[13,14] The test is a qualitative assay for the urease enzyme. The concepts underlying the test are straightforward, as are the factors that could lead to false-positive or false-negative results. Stool *H pylori* antigen testing is another method to assess the presence of an active *H pylori* infection, and although it is slightly less reliable compared to the UBT, it is also widely available.[15]

Stool Tests

Culture of *H pylori* from stool samples is difficult, and improved methods are needed. Recently, there has been increased interest in identifying *H pylori* protein antigens in stool as a marker of infection. Premier Platinum HpSA (Meridian Diagnostics Inc., Cincinnati, OH) has developed an in vitro qualitative enzyme immunoassay commercial kit that is stated to be able to detect *H pylori* protein antigens of concentration ≥184 ng/mL of feces. Overall, studies using pretreatment stool *H pylori* antigen tests have shown that the sensitivity and specificity of stool antigen testing was comparable to histology or urea breath testing. There is considerable lot-to-lot variation in stool antigen tests. The most likely explanation is that the polyclonal sera used for the capture antibody is obtained from rabbits and is thus difficult, if not impossible, to standardize. Stool antigen testing has proven to be less reliable when used soon after the end of therapy, and it is now generally recommended that one wait 6 or 8 weeks after therapy when using the stool antigen test to confirm eradication.[15] The UBT is preferred where available.

Urea Breath Testing

The UBT is the noninvasive method of choice to determine *H pylori* status (Figure 9). This test is based on the urease activity of the organism, splitting CO_2 from ingested urea. Ingestion of labeled urea allows the labeled CO_2 produced in this reaction to be detected in the breath. Two forms are available: the radioactive isotope of carbon ^{14}C and the stable, nonradioactive ^{13}C.

Radioactive substrate: ^{14}C-urea is ingested in a capsule, and breath samples are collected for detection of the $^{14}CO_2$. This can be done locally using the nuclear medicine department's equipment or sent to a central laboratory for

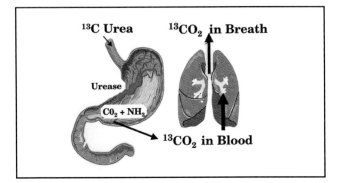

Figure 9: The urea breath test takes advantage of the high urease activity of *Helicobacter pylori*. Hydrolysis of labeled urea results in absorption of the labeled CO_2, which can be captured in the breath and analyzed. The urea breath test is the most efficient and accurate method to detect active *H pylori* infection and is especially suited for evaluation of the success of therapy.

analysis. The ^{14}C-urea breath test is inexpensive, but the use of radioactive compounds entails special licensing, and the staff performing these tests requires training in the use of radioactive chemicals. Although the amount of radioactivity is described as low, zero radioactive exposure is best, especially when nonradioactive testing is available.

Nonradioactive (stable isotope) urea: The Meretek UBT BreathTek™ (Meretek Diagnostics, Figure 10) uses the stable isotope of carbon, [13]C. The original test has been simplified and improved. The original test administered the urea after consumption of a test meal to prolong retention of the urea in the stomach. The current version uses citric acid as the test meal, allowing the urea and the test meal to be administered together. Fasting from solid food is only required for 1 hour. Exhaled breath is sampled before and 15 minutes after urea in-

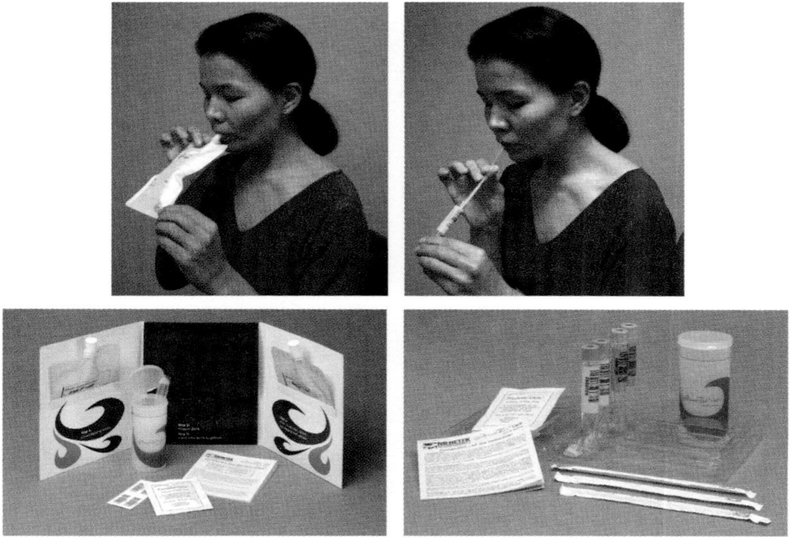

Figure 10: In the United States, the urea breath test is available in two versions. Both contain 75 mg of ^{13}C-urea and citric acid. One uses a breath collection bag; in the other, the individual collects the breath sample directly into the tube used for shipping the sample for analysis. The breath sample from the version that uses the bag is analyzed 'near patient' with an office-based infrared ^{13}CO$_2$ analyzer.

gestion. The breath samples are collected in a foil composite bag or test tube, depending on whether the test will be analyzed in the physician's office or sent to an outside laboratory. The bag is used with an infrared $^{13}CO_2$ analyzer (Figure 11), whereas the breath-filled tubes are sent to a central laboratory for processing. Results are available almost immediately when using the infrared analyzer and the next day for those samples that are sent out. Mass spectrophotometry and measurement of $^{13}CO_2/^{12}CO_2$ ratios directly using infrared spectroscopy provide equivalent results. For example, we compared the results of the UBiT®-IR300 and gas isotope ratio mass spectroscopy among 322 individuals: 64 patients were tested in an experienced laboratory and 258 in primary or secondary care clinics. There were 116 positive cases and 204 negative cases. Two cases were excluded from the analysis because one test was missing. The overall agreement between the two methods was 99.1%. The positive agreement was 98.3% (2 discordant); the negative agreement was 99.1% (1 discordant case). The overall relationship between the actual values measured was nearly linear (R=0.999). The availability of in-the-office urea breath testing should make the test the gold standard for diagnosis and for confirmation of success of therapy.

Because the ^{13}C-urea breath test involves no radiation, no special handling of the specimens is required. Also, pregnant women and children can be tested without concerns for safety, and repetitive testing poses no problems. The test can easily be performed in the physician's office.

Benefits and limitations of UBT methods: The UBT has a high sensitivity and specificity for the detection of active *H pylori* infection. Sensitivities are typically in the 95% range, with specificities of 95% to 100%.[16] These methods are simple to perform and are relatively inexpensive. No special handling of the ^{13}C-based test is required. Although the urea has no side effects, UBTs have some limitations and some decided advantages. The UBT,

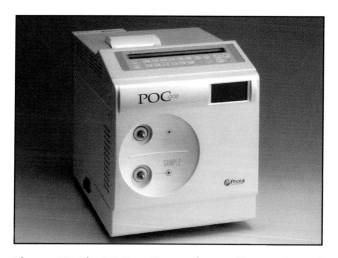

Figure 11: The POCone™, manufactured by Otsuka and distributed by Meretek, is commercially available throughout the United States.

like histology or urease testing, requires a high density of bacteria. The advantage of the UBT is that it is a 'global' assessment of the *H pylori* content of the stomach, whereas the other methods do not sample the entire gastric mucosa but test only the tiny biopsy specimen. Theoretically and practically, the UBT is the best method for detection of active *H pylori* infection. By convention, the UBT should not be conducted until 4 weeks after anti-*Helico-bacter* antibiotic therapy to allow any residual bacteria to increase to a number sufficient for detection. Any drug that diminishes *H pylori* numbers to below the threshold of detection can cause false-negative tests, particularly recent use of PPIs, bismuth-containing compounds, or antibiotics. These same cautions hold for all the methods that require the actual presence of bacteria. We recently confirmed our prior experience showing that false-negative UBT results occur in up to 40% of individuals taking PPIs. In that study, we investigated whether a citric acid test meal would prevent false-negative UBT results. Thirty *H pylori*-infected individuals underwent UBT with a citric acid test meal (BreathTek™ UBT) and then received omeprazole (Prilosec®) 20 mg twice daily for 13 days. UBTs were repeated after 6.5 days of PPI and 1, 2, 4, 7, and 14 days after PPI. Then, in a separate experiment, 9 of the original volunteers were rechallenged with omeprazole for 6.5 days. Antral and corpus biopsies for histology and culture were done before and 1 day after PPIs. Ten of the 30 *H pylori*-infected subjects developed transient negative UBT results; 9 after 6.5 days and nine 24 hours after ending the therapy. The result remained negative 1 day after ending PPI therapy in 6. After 2 days, the test was negative in only 1, which reverted to positive by day 14. Three of the 9 subjects who received a second omeprazole challenge developed transiently negative UBT results. In all 9, the *H pylori* density decreased in the antrum and corpus during PPI therapy. In many cases, the histology did not show any *H pylori*. These results confirmed our prior studies that false-negative UBT with PPI therapy reflects a transient reduction in *H pylori* load and not a redistribution of *H pylori* within the stomach. False-negative *H pylori* tests are not limited to the UBT but include all tests that reflect *H pylori* density (culture, histology, RUT, stool antigen). Because the UBT result reflects current actual intragastric *H pylori* load, it is affected the least and for the shortest time by PPI therapy.

Use of the UBT: The UBT is ideal when the question is whether the patient has an active *H pylori* infection. The test can be used to diagnose the infection before therapy, as well as to ascertain whether therapy has been successful. The UBT is the most economical, noninvasive, rapid, office-based technique to evaluate *H pylori* status. It should generally be the test of choice to confirm eradication of the infection after therapy (see below).

Table 2: Alarms or 'Red Flags' Prompting Endoscopy for the Evaluation of Patients with Dyspepsia

- Anemia
- Gastrointestinal bleeding
- Significant vomiting
- Anorexia with weight loss
- Presence of a mass
- Upper GI radiographic study with equivocal results

New Testing Methods

Molecular techniques are increasingly being applied in clinical medicine, particularly polymerase chain reaction tests (PCR). *H pylori* detection is no exception. In general, the specificity of PCR has been high, but the sensitivity has varied. Because of the technical difficulties, the presence of inhibitors, false-positive tests, and the excellent simple methods for traditional detection for *H pylori*, we believe that PCR will remain a research tool without any advantages over current noninvasive tests for *H pylori* detection.

When to Test for *Helicobacter pylori*

Confirmation of active *H pylori* infection should always prompt treatment.[17] The general rule 'do not test unless you are prepared to treat' is valid, and should be the basis for testing. No one wants, needs, or deserves an *H pylori* infection. Nevertheless, the infection is extremely common, and therapies are difficult. The primary indication to test is to identify an *H pylori* infection as the cause of a clinical problem or to prevent development of a disease (eg, peptic ulcer, gastric cancer). The typical indication for testing is dyspepsia, the presence or history of a peptic ulcer, or a family history of gastric cancer.[18,19]

Classic Peptic Symptoms

One of the most common settings for the question of whether to test for *H pylori* is when a patient presents with dyspepsia suggestive of peptic ulcer disease. These classic symptoms include epigastric pain, often described as burning and sharp. Patients frequently complain of accompanying abdominal discomfort or nausea. Symptoms may occur within 3 hours after a meal and may interrupt sleep. The symptoms typically occur on an empty stomach and are relieved by the intake of food or the use of antacids. The duration of symptoms in uncomplicated ulcer disease is months to years, waxing and waning over that time. Patients who smoke typically have prolonged courses, and many patients will report self-medication with over-the-counter antacids or with nonprescription H_2-receptor antagonists or PPIs.

Many patients with peptic ulcer will have been previously diagnosed with ulcer disease, by endoscopy or by barium meal studies. The approach to these patients is simple: test, treat, and evaluate the result of therapy.

The patient presenting with dyspepsia without a confirmed diagnosis presents a more difficult problem. An estimated 25% to 40% of the adult US population suffers at some time from dyspepsia. While recent estimates have revised that figure downward to the 13% range, 1% of a family physician's pool of patients can be expected to visit each year for new-onset dyspepsia. The symptoms are variable, although they typically fall into two groups: epigastric burning relieved by food or indigestion-predominant complaints.[20] Any group of patients with dyspepsia will contain patients with peptic ulcer, gastroesophageal reflux disease, and nonulcer dyspepsia. The approach to these patients is evolving. In 1996, the Practice Parameters Committee of the American College of Gastroenterology published guidelines that address the dyspeptic patient.[21] Three options are presented for evaluating and treating dyspeptic patients. The first involves empiric ulcer treatment with a short course (2 weeks) of antisecretory medication. A second option is immediate definitive diagnosis with endoscopy, which would be prudent if any warning signs were present. The third choice is noninvasive testing for *H pylori*.

The use of an anti-*Helicobacter* regimen without a definite diagnosis of *H pylori* infection is inappropriate. We believe that the approach should be to perform a history and physical examination and screening laboratory tests (eg, blood count and fecal blood testing). The goal is to identify those patients with alarming symptoms in whom early endoscopy is indicated (Table 2). While patients with gastroesophageal reflux disease may not immediately benefit from therapy for *H pylori*, peptic ulcer caused by *H pylori* infection can be cured. Nonetheless, patients with gastroesophageal reflux disease frequently receive long-term therapy with antisecretory drugs, especially PPIs. It has been demonstrated that such therapy removes the acid-associated 'protection' of the gastric corpus from *H pylori*-induced inflammation. As a consequence, the rate of development and the severity of corpus gastritis are accelerated. While it is not proven that this will increase the risk for the development of gastric cancer, it does increase the rate of development of the precursor lesion. Thus, consideration for long-term antisecretory therapy has joined the list of indications for testing for the presence of an *H pylori* infection.

Typical symptoms of gastroesophageal reflux disease are substernal discomfort (heartburn) exacerbated by lying flat, spicy food, or citrus drinks. Patients may experience regurgitation of gastric contents when supine. These patients can usually be identified by history alone. In contrast, it may be impossible to distinguish peptic ulcer from nonulcer dyspepsia. The link between *H pylori* infection and nonulcer dyspepsia is weak, and antibiotic therapy has not been consistently associated with symptom relief.

Table 3: Recommendations for Testing for *Helicobacter pylori* Infection

Definite

- Duodenal or gastric ulcer, active or history of
- Gastric MALT lymphoma
- Presence of atrophic gastritis
- Relatives of gastric cancer patients
- After endoscopic resection of early gastric cancer
- Uninvestigated dyspepsia
- Evaluate success of eradication therapy

Strongly recommended

- Nonulcer dyspepsia
- Plan chronic NSAID/aspirin therapy*
- Plan for chronic antisecretory drug therapy (eg, gastroesophageal reflux disease)**
- Relatives of patients with duodenal ulcer
- Relatives of patients with *H pylori* infection
- Patient desires to be tested

* When planning long-term therapy
** When planning long-term antisecretory therapy

Whom to Test for *Helicobacter pylori*

The wide variety of tests available for detection of *H pylori* has led to some confusion regarding which test to use, and when. It is important to know what to do with the results of a positive test before ordering the test. We believe that testing should not be done unless the clinician is willing to treat patients who test positive for the infection.[17,22] The recognition that *H pylori* causes a serious chronic and transmissible infection has led to an increase in the indications for testing (Table 3).

Diagnostic endoscopy is becoming reserved for those with complicated peptic ulcer, presence of alarming symptoms, and long-standing gastroesophageal reflux disease (to exclude Barrett's esophagus). Because of the high sensitivity, specificity, and rapidity of results, RUT is an excellent initial test of biopsy samples. If the patient has a high pretest probability (eg, a duodenal ulcer) and the RUT is positive and culture is not available, no further testing is required.[23] If the RUT is negative, then histologic examination of biopsy samples should be conducted. Culture is only necessary if antibiotic resistance profiles are required.

For those patients in whom endoscopy is not needed, serology, the UBT, or stool antigen testing is appropriate as a first diagnostic test, especially for patients not previously treated for *H pylori* infection. Positive serologic tests should be confirmed unless the pretest probability is high (eg, active duodenal ulcer). If the pretest probability is high and the serologic test is negative, a UBT or stool antigen test should be performed. Active *H pylori* infection should prompt treatment.

References

1.   Hachem CY, Clarridge JE, Evans DG, et al: Comparison of agar based media for primary isolation of *Helicobacter pylori*. *J Clin Pathol* 1995;48:714-716.

2.   Han SW, Flamm R, Hachem CY, et al: Transport and storage of *Helicobacter pylori* from gastric mucosal biopsies and clinical isolates. *Eur J Clin Microbiol Infect Dis* 1995;14:349-352.

3.   Ota H, Genta RM: Morphological characterization of the gastric mucosa during infection with *H pylori*. In: Ernst PB, Michetti P, Smith PD, eds. *The Immunobiology of* H pylori: *From Pathogenesis to Prevention*. Philadelphia, Lippincott-Raven, 1997, pp 15-28.

4.   Genta RM, Robason GO, Graham DY: Simultaneous visualization of *Helicobacter pylori* and gastric morphology: a new stain. *Hum Pathol* 1994;25:221-226.

5.   El-Zimaity HM, Wu, J, Graham DY: Modified Genta triple stain for identifying *Helicobacter pylori*. *J Clin Pathol* 1999;52: 693-694.

6.   El-Zimaity HM, Segura AM, Genta RM, et al: Histologic assessment of *Helicobacter pylori* status after therapy: comparison of Giemsa, Diff-Quik, and Genta stains. *Mod Pathol* 1998;11: 288-291.

7.   El-Zimaity HM, Wu J, Akamatsu T, et al: A reliable method for the simultaneous identification of *H pylori* and gastric metaplasia in the duodenum. *J Clin Pathol* 1999;52:914-916.

8.   Alpert LC, Graham DY, Evans DJ Jr, et al: Diagnostic possibilities for *Campylobacter pylori* infection. *Eur J Gastroenterol Hepatol* 1989;1:17-26.

9.   Dixon MF, Genta RM, Yardley JH, et al: Classification and grading of gastritis. The updated Sydney System. International Workshop on the Histopathology of Gastritis, Houston 1994. *Am J Surg Pathol* 1996;20:1161-1181.

10.   Blecker U, Vandenplas Y: Usefulness of specific IgM in the diagnosis of *Helicobacter pylori* infection. *Pediatrics* 1994; 93:342-343.

11.   Simor AE, Lin E, Saibil F, et al: Evaluation of enzyme immunoassay for detection of salivary antibody to *Helicobacter pylori*. *J Clin Microbiol* 1996;34:550-553.

12.   Graham DY, Reddy S: Rapid detection of anti-*Helicobacter pylori* IgG in urine using immunochromatography. *Aliment Pharmacol Ther* 2001;15:699-702.

13.   Graham DY, Malaty HM, Cole RA, et al: Simplified ^{13}C-urea breath test for detection of *Helicobacter pylori* infection. *Am J Gastroenterol* 2001;96:1741-1745.

14.   Graham DY, Klein PD: Accurate diagnosis of *Helicobacter pylori*. ^{13}C-urea breath test. *Gastroenterol Clin North Am* 2000;29:885-893.

15.   Graham DY, Qureshi WA: Markers of infection. In: Mobley HL, Mendz GL, Hazell SL, eds. *Helicobacter pylori: Physiology and Genetics*. Washington, DC, ASM Press, 2001, pp 499-510.

16.   Klein PD, Malaty HM, Martin RF, et al: Noninvasive detection of *Helicobacter pylori* infection in clinical practice: the ^{13}C urea breath test. *Am J Gastroenterol* 1996;91:690-694.

17.   Rabeneck L, Graham DY: *Helicobacter pylori*: when to test, when to treat. *Ann Intern Med* 1997;126:315-316.

18.   Nakajima S, Graham DY, Hattori T, et al: Strategy for treatment of *Helicobacter pylori* infection in adults. I. Updated indications for test and eradication therapy suggested in 2000. *Curr Pharm Des* 2000;6:1503-1514.

19.   Miehlke S, Bayerdorffer E, Graham DY: Treatment of *Helicobacter pylori* infection. *Semin Gastrointest Dis* 2001;12: 167-179.

20.   Ofman JJ, Etchason J, Fullerton S, et al: Management strategies for *Helicobacter pylori*-seropositive patients with dyspepsia: clinical and economic consequences. *Ann Intern Med* 1997; 126:280-291.

21.   Soll AH: Consensus conference. Medical treatment of peptic ulcer disease. Practice guidelines. Practice Parameters Committee of the American College of Gastroenterology. *JAMA* 1996;275: 622-629.

22.   Graham DY: Can therapy ever be denied for *Helicobacter pylori* infection? *Gastroenterology* 1997;113:S113-S117.

23.   Peura DA: *Helicobacter pylori*: a diagnostic dilemma and a dilemma of diagnosis. *Gastroenterology* 1995;109:313-315.

Chapter **6**

Therapy

Throughout much of the 20th century, the dictum 'no acid, no ulcer' was invoked as important in the pathogenesis of peptic ulcer; exceptions were few. The discovery that *Helicobacter pylori* had a major role in the pathogenesis of ulcer led to the dictum 'no *H pylori* infection, no ulcer.' This conceptual change ushered in the era of antibiotic treatment of ulcer disease. Although acid is still important in ulcerogenesis, establishing that the cure of the bacterial infection results in cure of ulcer disease changed thinking and therapy[1] (Figure 1).

H pylori infection is not cured easily, and research has shown a need for multidrug therapy. Although many treatment regimens are clinically successful, simple, seemingly intuitive alterations in therapy have led to treatment failures. We still have little information about why some therapies fail, and until we better understand the different niches the bacterium may occupy, it is crucial to use a regimen tested in large populations and used 'as is' to have the highest chance of success.

Aims of Therapy

The aims of therapy for peptic ulcer disease are many. Cure of the *H pylori* infection is crucial. Patients come to doctors because of symptoms and for relief of symptoms, and healing active ulcers also is important. Both can be accomplished without curing the infection. Elimination of *H pylori* eliminates the need for maintenance antisecretory therapy for peptic ulcers, as well as for future physician visits for ulcer symptoms. Cure of the disease also prevents

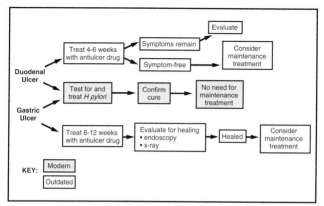

Figure 1: The modern-era *Helicobacter pylori* approach contrasted to the previous antisecretory-therapy approach to peptic ulcer disease. The new approach stresses therapy based on the etiology of the ulcer disease and is predicated on ability to cure the disease and to prevent new ulcers.

ulcer complications. Finally, therapy should be tailored to reduce or eliminate treatment-related complications and to minimize development of bacterial resistance.

An ideal therapy might have the following characteristics: low cost, high rate of treatment success, simplicity of administration, good tolerability, and few side effects. Although no current therapy meets all these criteria, a number of therapies are effective and well tolerated.

Agents Used in Therapy of Ulcers Caused by *Helicobacter pylori* Infection

The three broad categories of drugs used in treatment regimens for acid-peptic diseases associated with *H pylori* infection include antacids, antisecretory agents, and antimicrobial drugs. Antacids were the main agents in treating peptic disease until H_2-receptor antagonists became available. Popular antacids include Maalox®,

Tums®, Mylanta®, and Alka-Seltzer®. These agents provide quick pain relief for patients with symptomatic ulcer disease and are available without a prescription. H_2-Receptor antagonists and proton pump inhibitors (PPIs) have largely made antacid therapy obsolete for treatment of peptic ulcer disease.

Antisecretory Agents

Antisecretory agents accelerate the healing of ulcers regardless of etiology and can be considered 'healing agents.' Similar to antacids, they also relieve ulcer-associated discomfort and are safe.

H_2-Receptor antagonists: H_2-Receptor antagonists are widely used antisecretory agents. They are competitively reversible inhibitors of histamine at the H_2-receptor on the parietal cell. Available drugs are equally efficacious and safe and differ primarily in potency. Available drugs include cimetidine (Tagamet®), ranitidine (Zantac®), famotidine (Pepcid®), and nizatidine (Axid®). These drugs have been licensed for sale over the counter, usually at reduced dosages, including Tagamet HB®, Zantac 75®, Pepcid AC®, and Axid®, below those typically used in anti-*H pylori* regimens. H_2-Receptor antagonists have no antibacterial activity against *H pylori*.

Proton pump inhibitors: PPIs block acid secretion at the hydrogen-potassium ATPase pump on the luminal border of the gastric parietal cell. This pump exchanges hydrogen for potassium across the parietal cell microvillus membrane, secreting hydrogen ions into the gastric lumen and creating the low-pH environment characteristic of gastric secretions. PPIs bind and inhibit ATPase, increasing the intraluminal gastric pH. PPIs are the most effective antisecretory agents, achieving better pH control than H_2-receptor antagonists. Available agents include omeprazole (Prilosec®), lansoprazole (Prevacid®), pantoprazole (Protonix®), rabeprazole (Aciphex®), and esomeprazole (Nexium®). The PPIs have direct antibacterial activity against *H pylori* but when used alone will not cure the infection. As stated in the chapter on diagnosis, PPI therapy reduces the *H pylori* load in the stomach and can result in negative diagnostic test results.

Anticholinergics: Anticholinergic agents have weak antisecretory ability and no antibacterial activity against *H pylori*, and they should be considered obsolete for treatment of ulcer disease.

Prostaglandins: The synthetic prostaglandin misoprostol (Cytotec®) is useful for prevention of ulcers caused by nonsteroidal anti-inflammatory drugs (NSAIDs). Misoprostol is a synthetic prostaglandin E_1, and although it has FDA approval for prophylaxis against peptic ulceration in patients using NSAIDs, it has no antimicrobial activity against *H pylori* and has not been shown to have a role in *H pylori* therapy.

Sucralfate: Sucralfate (Carafate®) is a topical antiulcer drug. Sucralfate is the aluminum hydroxide salt of sulfated sucrose. Its main activity is coating of ulcer sites, leading to slightly increased rates of ulcer healing. It does have an effect on *H pylori* adherence in vitro, but has not demonstrated any convincing anti-*H pylori* effect in vitro. It is generally considered obsolete for treatment of ulcer disease. It has no effect on NSAID ulcers.

Antimicrobials

H pylori is a bacterial infection of a mucosal surface. As with other bacterial infections, the mainstay of therapy is antimicrobials to which the bacterium is sensitive. Because the infection is inside the stomach but outside the body (intraluminal), there may be a place for topical therapy. In fact, because of the hostile acid environment of the stomach, topical therapy may greatly enhance overall effectiveness. It is not clear how much of the efficacy of current therapies is related to the topical action of the drugs and how much is attributable to systemic action, but both probably are important. Considerable evidence suggests that *H pylori* can invade surface epithelial cells. Thus, the combination of topical and systemic actions may be best (Table 1).

Table 1: Combination Therapies

Proton pump inhibitor triple therapy

Proton pump inhibitor at standard doses twice daily plus two of the three antibiotics given twice a day:

- Amoxicillin: 1 g
- Clarithromycin: 500 mg
- Metronidazole: 500 mg

Traditional triple therapy given four times daily

- Bismuth subsalicylate: two tablets
- Metronidazole: 250 or 500 mg
- Tetracycline HCl: 500 mg
- Antisecretory drug: (once daily)

Quadruple therapy

- Bismuth subsalicylate or citrate: two tablets four times daily
- Metronidazole: 500 mg three times daily
- Tetracycline HCl: 500 mg four times daily
- Proton pump inhibitor twice daily

Topical agents: Bismuth salts have been used to treat gastritis and peptic ulcers for more than 200 years.[2] For example, the antibacterial activity of bismuth resulted in its use to treat syphilis before modern antibiotics became available. Bismuth also has been used to prevent *Escherichia coli* traveler's diarrhea based on the antimicrobial activity of bismuth salts.[3] Bismuth is directly bactericidal to *H pylori* and leads to bacterial lysis. Ultrastructural examination shows precipitation of bismuth around *H pylori* organisms, followed by accumulation beneath the bacterial cell wall, detachment of the organism from the mucosa, and bacterial lysis, all within 2 hours of ingestion.[4] On ingesting bismuth, there is an immediate and marked reduction in bacterial numbers, thereby reducing the chance a colony resistant to antibiotics will survive (see below). *H pylori* does not develop resistance to the various bismuth salts, which may make bismuth an important component of *H pylori* therapy in the future. One form of bismuth, the colloid suspension of bismuth citrate, also coats the ulcer and encourages ulcer healing. There is no evidence that bismuth subsalicylate has this coating effect, yet it is an effective anti-*H pylori* agent.[5]

Bismuth has an excellent safety record; the most troublesome side effects are temporary discoloration of the tongue and development of black stools. There is a hypothetical concern about systemic absorption of bismuth leading to bismuth toxicity, but this has not been a clinical problem. However, if the common subsalicylate form of bismuth is used, significant salicylate ingestion will occur. For example, each tablet of Pepto-Bismol® contains 225 mg of salicylate, and most is absorbed. Patients receiving salicylate therapy should have their doses modified, and patients who should avoid salicylates (eg, children younger than 16 years) should consider an alternate form of bismuth. In the United States, bismuth is available as bismuth subsalicylate (Pepto-Bismol®). Ranitidine bismuth citrate (Tritec®, Pylorid®) is available in many countries but is no longer available in the United States because it did not achieve sufficient sales, not because it was ineffective.

Traditional Antimicrobials

H pylori is sensitive to many different antibiotics, and a variety of antibiotics and antibiotic combinations has been tried. The antibiotics that have proven effective include clarithromycin (Biaxin®), amoxicillin, metronidazole (Flagyl®, Protostat®), tetracycline, and furazolidone (Furoxone®) (Table 2). Cure rates with single antibiotic agents have been poor, from 0% to 35%.[6] Monotherapy

Table 2: Antimicrobial Agents Available in the United States and Proven Useful for Treatment of *Helicobacter pylori* Infection

- Amoxicillin
- Bismuth
- Clarithromycin (Biaxin®)
- Metronidazole (Flagyl®, Protostat®)
- Tinidazole (Tindamax®)
- Tetracycline
- Furazolidone (Furoxone®)
- Fluoroquinolones
- Proton pump inhibitors

is associated with the rapid development of antibiotic resistance, especially to metronidazole and clarithromycin.

Many physicians have attempted to modify established protocols by using another antibiotic in the same class, such as substitution of azithromycin (Zithromax®) for clarithromycin or doxycycline for tetracycline. With the exception of tinidazole (Tindamax®), which can be used interchangeably with metronidazole, substitutions have led to markedly lower efficacy and are not recommended.

Clarithromycin: Clarithromycin is a macrolide that binds to bacterial ribosomes and disrupts protein synthesis, leading to bacterial cell death. Clarithromycin is the most acid-stable of the macrolides and has the lowest minimum inhibitory concentration (MIC). The chief metabolite of clarithromycin also is active against *H pylori*. Like other monotherapies, clarithromycin alone yields poor results. Administration with a PPI greatly increases the area under the curve and results in 2-fold higher concentrations of clarithromycin in the antral mucosa and 10-fold higher levels in the mucus layer.[6,7] Clarithromycin is generally well tolerated. Reported side effects include an altered sense of taste, frequently described as metallic; nausea; vomiting; and headache. Drug interactions between this class of antibiotics (macrolides) and antihistamines are important, specifically terfenadine (Seldane®, removed from the market in 1997) and astemizole (Hismanal®), as well as cisapride (Propulsid®, no longer marketed in the United States), and they have been associated with cardiac arrhythmias and death. Clarithromycin also increases theophylline and carbamazepine levels. Clarithromycin resistance is increasing; resistance predicts treatment failure.

Amoxicillin: Amoxicillin is an acid-stable semisynthetic penicillin that is bactericidal in vivo. The antimicrobial activity of amoxicillin is pH dependent; MIC decreases as pH increases. Resistance to amoxicillin is rare but has been reported and may be partly responsible for the markedly variable success of the combination of a PPI and amoxicillin. Amoxicillin concentrations are highest in the antral mucosa; lower levels are achieved in the corpus mucosa and the mucus layer. Overall, results with combination therapy that includes amoxicillin have been good, suggesting that sufficient levels are achieved and that it is an effective anti-*H pylori* agent when used as part of a combination therapy.

Metronidazole: Metronidazole is a nitroimidazole that is selectively toxic to microaerophilic microorganisms. Metronidazole is a prodrug, and a chemically reactive, reduced form of the drug leads to generation of cytotoxic products and destruction of microorganisms. The activity of metronidazole is largely independent of pH, making it theoretically ideal for the gastric environment. Unfortunately, *H pylori* rapidly develops resistance to metronidazole, and the widespread use of this drug has resulted in high primary resistance. In the United States, primary resistance of *H pylori* to metronidazole ranges from 20% to

50%; in developing countries, resistance often is present in more than 70% of isolates. The mechanism of resistance is unclear, and several different pathways probably lead to the resistance phenotype. Metronidazole resistance identified in vitro does not always predict resistance in vivo; thus, this agent may remain useful despite a high level of resistance in a population or even in an individual (see below).

Tetracycline: Tetracycline hydrochloride was used in the first effective therapies against *H pylori* and remains an important antibiotic. The activity of tetracycline is independent of gastric acidity, making it potentially important. Tetracycline is inexpensive, and resistance is rare. Success has been reported with tetracycline hydrochloride and with oxytetracycline (Terramycin®), whereas doxycycline has produced inferior results. Tetracyclines are contraindicated in children because of the abnormal pigmentation of permanent dentition that occurs when the drug is used while teeth are being calcified.

Furazolidone: Furazolidone is a synthetic nitrofuran with broad antibacterial activity based on interference with bacterial enzymes. It has been used in China for treatment of peptic ulcers and is now widely used to treat *H pylori* infections in China and South America.[8,9] Resistance is rare, and even when present is low. Furazolidone has proven effective as part of triple-drug therapies and is especially useful in salvage therapies.[10,11] Furazolidone is a monoamine oxidase inhibitor, and the patient must be cautioned to avoid drug-drug and drug-food interactions. Foods to be avoided include aged cheese, sausage, bologna, salami and pepperoni, lima beans, lentils, snow peas, and soybeans, canned figs and raisins, all alcoholic beverages, natural licorice, and any food product that is made with soy sauce. Drugs to be avoided include all other monoamine oxidase inhibitors, isocarboxazid (Marplan®), phenelzine (Nardil™), tranylcypromine (Parnate™), and common cold remedies and over-the-counter allergy medications that contain phenylpropanolamine, ephedrine, or phenylephrine.

Rifabutin: Rifabutin (Mycobutin®) is a derivative of rifampin and a semisynthetic ansamycin antibiotic with a very low MIC level for *H pylori*. Because of its high lipophilicity, rifabutin has a high propensity for distribution and intracellular tissue uptake. Rifabutin is believed to inhibit DNA-dependent RNA polymerase, resulting in impaired growth and protein synthesis. It is used extensively in the treatment of *Mycobacterium avium* complex disease with advanced HIV infection. Rifabutin-based rescue therapy constitutes an encouraging strategy after multiple previous eradication failures with key antibiotics such as amoxicillin, clarithromycin, metronidazole, and tetracycline.[10,12] Side effects from rifabutin include upset stomach, stomach cramps, nausea, headache, rash, neutropenia, and altered taste.

Fluoroquinolones: Fluoroquinolones have been used successfully. Moxifloxacin (Avelox®), levofloxacin (Levaquin®), and gatifloxacin (Tequin®) appear to give better results than ciprofloxacin (Cipro®), despite comparable in vitro activity. Quinolones block DNA gyrase and inhibit DNA synthesis. Resistance occurs by a point mutation in the gyrase A protein.[13,14] Resistance develops rapidly such that quinolones should only be used as a component of combination therapy. The widespread use of these drugs for other infections will likely lead to widespread resistance and limit their usefulness. Use is limited in patients younger than 18 years and in women who are pregnant or breastfeeding. Caution should be used in patients with risk factors for QT(c) prolongation or disorders that predispose them to seizures, and in diabetic patients receiving concomitant antihyperglycemic agents. Caution is also required when administering concurrently with theophylline, warfarin, NSAIDs, and drugs reducing potassium and magnesium. Antacids, iron preparations, and sucralfate should not be taken within 2 hours of administration. In contrast with other fluoroquinolones, moxifloxacin is associated with fewer phototoxic and central nervous system excitatory effects and does not seem to interact with theophylline, warfarin, probenecid, and ranitidine. The most common adverse events of moxifloxacin are gastrointestinal disturbances, such as nausea and diarrhea, because of the impact on the human intestinal microflora, mainly on the enterobacteria.

Investigational Agents

Besides the previously mentioned antibiotics, numerous other drugs are under investigation for treatment of *H pylori* infection. Ecabet, a Japanese antiulcer medicine, is undergoing trials. This agent has been shown to have some activity against *H pylori* in vitro, and when added to a regimen including lansoprazole and amoxicillin, cure rates increased from 58% to 78%. There is interest, but limited experience, with agents that may reduce the mucus barrier, such as pronase or acetylcysteine (Mucosil®), for improving the efficacy of traditional antibiotics. We look forward to the results of the many innovative experiments that are being done worldwide in the search for better, simpler therapies for *H pylori* infection.

Treatment Regimens

Many issues should be considered when selecting a regimen for treatment of *H pylori* infection. These include cost, simplicity, efficacy, side effects, community antibiotic resistance, dose, duration, frequency of administration, whether to administer with meals or fasting, and whether control of pH is needed.[15,16] The best therapy is one that reliably cures the infection. The worst and most expensive therapy is one that fails to cure the infection. A number of arbitrary 'rules' or goals for therapy have been published. Typically, an effective regimen must cure at least 90% of infections with no more than twice-daily therapy for no more than 7 days. Such thinking is unrealistic.

The amount of literature dedicated to *H pylori* treatment protocols is almost overwhelming. Hundreds of small clinical trials have been reported. Overall, they have confirmed that eradication of *H pylori* infection cures peptic ulcer disease and that reliable treatment of the infection is difficult. Conclusions often are based on studies involving 10 to 20 patients. Published meta-analyses have often included results obtained from abstracts involving small numbers of patients, rendering the conclusions suspect. Overall, the only consistency is that rates of success and details of drug administration vary widely.

Studies can be exploratory or confirmatory. Exploratory studies are designed to evaluate the efficacy of a new drug combination, a variation of a combination, or an established combination in a new population or different geographic region. Exploratory studies are generally small. As a rule of thumb, a sample size of at least 30 patients is required to establish reliable confidence intervals to allow for interpretation of the study.[17] The 95% confidence intervals yield more accurate estimates of the results that could be expected from clinical use of the regimen than does the percent cured. For example, if a study had a 90% cure rate, the 95% confidence intervals for a study with only 10 patients would have a broad range from 55% to 99%. For 50 subjects undergoing the same experiment, the confidence intervals would have a narrower range from, say, 78% to 96%; for 100 subjects, 82% to 95%; and for 200 patients, 85% to 94%.

Confirmatory studies are typically large, multicenter trials that test a therapy or therapies in different communities. These provide a better estimate of what physicians can expect. Confirmatory studies are required for reliable data on how to treat this disease.

Specific Treatment Regimens

The original highly successful therapy for eradicating *H pylori* was developed by Borody et al in 1989.[18] This regimen involved three drugs—bismuth, metronidazole, and tetracycline—and was labeled *BMT triple therapy*.

However, a number of different triple therapies have led to a profusion of abbreviations. Although these regimens have no standard nomenclature, the names are typically derived from the component drugs.[19] For example, 'BCT' triple therapy refers to bismuth, clarithromycin, and tetracycline. 'BMT-PPI' refers to Borody's combination with the addition of a PPI. Such terminology probably is needed to assist in distinguishing among the different regimens. However, it does not give details of dosage or duration; thus, the actual details must be reviewed before trying a specific combination that appears effective.

FDA-Approved Regimens

Because higher success rates can be achieved, triple-drug combinations are recommended. Worldwide, the most frequently prescribed therapy is a triple therapy consisting of a PPI and clarithromycin and amoxicillin. The typical therapy is to give a standard dose of the PPI, 500 mg of clarithromycin, and 1 g of amoxcillin twice a day for 7, 10, or 14 days. We recommend at least 10 days and prefer 14 days. The alternative therapy is to replace the 1 g of amoxicillin with 500 mg of metronidazole. There are no data to suggest that one PPI is superior to another with regard to *H pylori* eradication therapy (see later explanation). As noted previously, ranitidine bismuth citrate is no longer available in the United States, but studies in other countries have shown that it can replace the PPI in these twice-daily triple therapies.

Practical Issues Regarding Choices of Antimicrobial Regimens

An evidence-based choice of treatment regimen is nearly impossible because large randomized trials comparing the most effective regimens have rarely been done. Even the most effective regimens available fail in 20% to 40% of patients. For example, several meta-analyses have shown that with the most commonly used therapies, cure rates are typically less than 85%.[20-24] Although meta-analysis is usually a powerful tool in understanding the efficacy of treatment, it is less helpful in choosing the best therapy because of the presence of considerable heterogeneity in data, including absence of crucial data such as the presence/absence of pretreatment antimicrobial resistance. There are only a few head-to-head comparisons of different antibiotic dosages or duration of therapies, leaving the influence of these parameters on treatment success unknown. Finally, and unexpectedly, based on the response to treatment of other infectious diseases, the cure rates often differ greatly in different countries despite using the same regimen.[23,25]

Generally, a longer duration of treatment (eg, 14 days vs 7 days) increases the cure rate.[24,25] Unfortunately, duration of therapy has been used to obtain marketing advantages, so less-than-optimum durations are common. We recommend 14 days. Large population-based trials have also shown that the high rates of success expected from the pharmaceutical-company-sponsored trials are often unattainable in clinical practice. Examples of large trials include 1,161 patients, using the combination of a PPI (omeprazole, 20 mg twice a day), clarithromycin (250 mg b.i.d), and tinidazole (500 mg b.i.d), who achieved cure rates of only 61% (95% CI = 58% to 64%).[26] A study of 812 patients receiving a standard Maastricht Consensus PPI-based regimen (PPI plus amoxicillin and clarithromycin for 7 days) achieved a cure rate of 72% (95% CI = 69% to 75%),[27] and a study of 890 patients receiving a PPI plus amoxicillin and clarithromycin for 7 days had a cure rate of 77% (0.5% CI = 74% to 80%).[28] Clearly, physicians' and patients' expectations are not being met with regard to success of therapy, and therapy choice based on published pharmaceutical-company-sponsored trials in highly selected populations often provide a misleading estimate of effectiveness. Choice of therapy based on the results of susceptibility testing will yield the best results, but susceptibility testing is generally unavailable, forcing physicians to use other methods of choosing therapies and their order.

First-line Therapies

The most widely used first-line therapies to eradicate *H pylori* consist of a PPI or, where available, ranitidine bismuth citrate, and two antibiotics (clarithromycin plus amoxicillin or plus metronidazole). The most effective and best-tolerated combination seems to be a twice-a-day combination of 1,000 mg of amoxicillin and 500 mg of clarithromycin (PPI + AC) or 500 mg of metronidazole and either 250 or 500 mg of clarithromycin (PPI + MC). There are data suggesting that the lower dose of clarithromycin in the metronidazole-clarithromycin combination may be equally effective, and the lower dose is slightly better tolerated.[29] However, the higher dose has generally proven superior,[30] and in the United States, the cost of 250 and 500 mg of clarithromycin is the same, and most use the higher dose. Convenient dose packs are available in the United Sates (eg, Prevpac®, whose components include lansoprazole 30 mg twice a day, clarithromycin 500 mg twice a day, and amoxicillin 1,000 mg twice a day) (Table 3). An additional convenience is that often only one co-pay is required instead of three when the drugs are purchased separately. For children, triple therapy using a PPI plus two antibiotics (eg, omeprazole 1 mg/kg/day up to 20 mg twice a day or comparable PPI; clarithromycin 15 mg/kg/day up to 500 mg twice a day; and amoxicillin 50 mg/kg/day up to 1,000 mg twice a day, or metronidazole 20 mg/kg/day up to 500 mg twice a day) is also recommended as the initial treatment.[31]

All of the PPIs appear equally effective with the clarithromycin-amoxicillin or metronidazole triple therapies, and they can be used interchangeably depending on local availability and cost.[27,32] H_2-Receptor antagonists are also effective, but the only benefit is a slight reduction in cost of therapy.[33] Healing rates and time to pain relief are better with PPIs and they are generally preferred. The minimal duration is 7 days, but as discussed above, this duration was not chosen based on multiple head-to-head

**Table 3: Convenience Dose Packs
Available in the United States**

Prevpac® components:

1. Lansoprazole (Prevacid®), 30 mg PO b.i.d.

2. Clarithromycin, 500 mg PO b.i.d.

3. Amoxicillin, 1,000 mg PO b.i.d.

Helidac® triple therapy components:

1. Bismuth subsalicylate, 525 mg (two 262.4-mg chewable tablets) (q.i.d.)

2. Metronidazole, 250 mg (q.i.d.)

3. Tetracycline hydrochloride, 500 mg (q.i.d.)

comparison and typically results are better with longer durations of therapy.[25] The optimum duration is unknown.

The original effective therapy was a combination of bismuth, metronidazole, and tetracycline (BMT) with an antisecretory drug. All of the antimicrobial drugs were off-patent and were pH independent. Being off-patent resulted in little interest among pharmaceutical companies. The original doses were tetracycline 500 mg, metronidazole 250 mg, and two bismuth tablets all given four times daily, generally for 14 days. A version of the original bismuth metronidazole tetracycline triple therapy is available as a dose pack (Helidac®) and is designed for 14 days of therapy along with an antisecretory drug (H_2-receptor antagonist or PPI). It is relatively inexpensive and remains popular in the United States (Table 3).

Second-Line Therapy

Second-line therapy is given after the initial therapy has failed. As mentioned previously, the best results are attained by choices based on the results of susceptibility testing, but because they are unavailable, the regimen is chosen based on using drugs that have not been administered previously.[34,35] Typically, quadruple therapy is recommended after triple therapies have failed to eradicate the *H pylori* infection.[36,37] Quadruple therapy is based on the BMT triple therapy. The changes are the addition of a PPI and a higher dose of metronidazole (from 250 mg four times daily to 500 mg three times daily). This combination has proven effective even with metronidazole resistance.[38,39] Despite the large number of tablets and the frequent drug administrations, dropout rates in most clinical trials have been comparable to those of easier twice a day triple-therapy regimens, and compliance has not proven to be a clinically important issue. Unfortunately, the literature is full of papers on different combinations called quadruple therapy, resulting in confusion among physicians and those doing meta-analyses. As quadruple therapy also uses off-patent antibiotics, it is more often a target for marketing studies rather than for scientific comparisons. An example is the recent pharmaceutical-company-supported multicenter QUADRATE study, which compared a traditional PPI, clarithromycin, and amoxicillin triple therapy with a suboptimum quadruple regimen.[40]

Is pH Control Needed as an Adjuvant to Antimicrobial Therapy?

Many *H pylori* treatment regimens are complicated, requiring administration of many different drugs at multiple intervals. The complexity of such regimens has prompted the continuing search for simplified treatment protocols. Because triple-drug therapies seem necessary to achieve maximum cure rates, twice-daily drug administrations and reductions in the duration of therapy have been attempted. Most twice-daily protocols have used a PPI given once or twice a day. PPIs have several potential benefits over H_2-receptor antagonists, including better pH control, more rapid pain relief, and an inherent antimicrobial action against *H pylori*.[6] Nevertheless, it is important to note that head-to-head comparisons of PPIs and H_2-receptor antagonists as adjuvants to antimicrobial therapy suggest that PPIs and H_2-receptor antagonists may be equivalent with respect to the antisecretory drug in combination with amoxicillin and either clarithromycin or metronidazole. In contrast, there seems to be a slight advantage for the PPI when the combination is an antisecretory drug, amoxicillin, and metronidazole.[41,42] Although head-to head comparison is the only method to answer whether PPIs have a significant advantage over H_2-receptor antagonists, there is little interest in the answer to this question because cost is the only feature that favors H_2-receptor antagonists. We believe that even if PPIs and H_2-receptor anagonists are equal, most clinicians would continue to use PPIs for these short-duration therapies because of their superior efficacy in pain relief, healing, pH control, etc. Although most published studies of PPIs in therapy of *H pylori* infection involve omeprazole, there is no reason to believe that omeprazole, lansoprazole, pantoprazole, rabeprazole, and esomeprazole are not interchangeable.

Proton Pump Inhibitor Triple and Quadruple Therapies

As noted above, the most common triple therapy worldwide is the twice-daily combination of clarithromycin (250 or 500 mg b.i.d.), metronidazole (500 mg b.i.d.), or amoxicillin 1 g and a PPI for 7 to 14 days.

The addition of a PPI to BMT triple therapy and an increase in the dose of metronidazole to 500 mg three times daily is called *BMT quadruple therapy*, and this combination seems to be the most reliable therapy.[6,43,44]

Some investigators have used furazolidone in place of metronidazole in bismuth triple therapy and quadruple therapy.[6,9] The most common dose is furazolidone 100 mg t.i.d. Furazolidone has been associated with nausea, vomiting, headache, tachycardia, and elevated blood pressure.

Furazolidone is a monoamine oxidase inhibitor and can interact with a number of other drugs and foods; therefore, dietary restrictions are required. In our experience, furazolidone drug combinations often are poorly tolerated, and we reserve them for salvage therapies. In the United States, furazolidone is expensive and difficult to obtain.

Administration Fasting or With Meals

The two important considerations in the stomach that can be easily influenced are gastric emptying and acidity. Administration of a drug to a fasting patient may result in most of the agent passing into the small intestine before the formulation can dissolve or disperse. The presence of food delays gastric emptying, is associated with excellent dispersion of an agent, and buffers gastric acid.[3,45] Administration with meals may prolong residence in the stomach, and the grinding and mixing functions of the stomach ensure wide drug dispersion. The practical aspects of the importance of administration of some drugs with meals is illustrated by the preliminary results obtained with ranitidine bismuth subcitrate combinations. Clearance and cure were significantly higher when the bismuth-containing preparation was given with meals, compared with fasting administration. One potentially negative aspect of administration with meals is that the drug may interact with components of the meal and become less available locally or for absorption. Finally, eating has the beneficial effect of causing desquamation of surface cells and discharge of mucus, which also possibly exposes the organisms to higher concentrations of the agent or exposes a higher percentage of the organisms to the agent.[46,47]

Antimicrobial action could possibly be improved by cotherapies with mucolytics or antisecretory drugs. Although there are few data on mucolytics, a number of studies have examined antimicrobial and antisecretory agents. The potential advantages of coadministration of antisecretory drugs include a decrease in intragastric volume (ie, increased antimicrobial concentration), increased intragastric pH (possibly increasing efficacy), and a possible direct antimicrobial effect of the antisecretory agent (eg, PPIs).

Duration of Therapy

The quest for simplified therapies has resulted in attempts to discover the shortest duration of antimicrobial therapy; numerous small, underpowered, uninterpretable studies have been published. The ramifications of these experiments have clearly not been examined, and, in our opinion, such efforts are possibly misguided. Shorter duration implies savings in costs for medications and potentially fewer side effects; it provides no other advantages and potentially increases the percentage of treatment failures.

The goal is to identify the optimal therapy, not the shortest. The steps in the development of a universally effective therapy probably should consist of identifying the best combination of drugs, doses, and dosing intervals. After the important details of the proposed therapy are established, we might then ask how the therapy could be further improved (eg, the optimum duration).

In many studies in the United States and Europe, the rank order of success is 14 days, which is superior to 10 days, which in turn is superior to 7 days.[48] Studies of the treatment of peptic ulcer from Europe have consistently yielded better healing (or cure) rates than those in the United States. Until head-to-head comparisons are available from multicenter trials that control for important variables, we recommend 14 days of therapy.

Treatment Failures

H pylori has proven difficult to cure. Some of the reasons for failure are easily understood, such as failure of the patient to take the antibiotics or the presence of antibiotic-resistant organisms. Some other potential causes of treatment failure are listed in Table 4. The association between treatment failure and other factors may differ among regimens. The dual therapy of a PPI plus amoxicillin proved very sensitive to external factors such as

Table 4: Possible Reasons for Treatment Failure

- Not taking the drugs (poor compliance)
- Resistance of the organism to the antibiotics
- Adverse drug interactions
- Poor distribution or concentration of antibiotic
  - antimicrobial unable to penetrate the site of the bacteria
  - anaerobic environment
  - presence of inactivating enzymes or binding proteins
  - biofilm phenomenon

smoking. Other hypotheses for poor results related to an adverse effect of pretreatment with PPIs and the type of underlying peptic disease. None of these factors predicts a poor result with the triple therapies.

Antibiotic Resistance

Resistance to antibiotics has increasingly been recognized as a worldwide problem. *H pylori* is no exception. Resistance to metronidazole and clarithromycin develops quickly, mandating the use of multidrug therapies. Resistance to antibiotics in *H pylori* has been chromosomally mediated and not plasmid mediated, even though plasmids can be detected in half of the isolates. Current practices do not include pretreatment culture and susceptibility determination. Experience has proven that if one course of therapy fails, the surviving organisms are or have become resistant to the key drug (eg, metronidazole or clarithromycin). Patients at high risk for harboring metronidazole-resistant organisms include women who may have received prior courses of metronidazole, immigrants from parts of the world with high rates of metronidazole resistance, and people from countries where metronidazole is available over the counter. Metronidazole resistance is poorly understood. A number of different enzymes within *H pylori* can activate the drug such that the presence of resistant strains does not preclude the use of metronidazole, although the success rates are expected to be lower.[49,50]

Clarithromycin resistance is a growing problem, although not yet as common as metronidazole resistance. Five percent to 14% of US isolates are resistant to clarithromycin. Resistance to one macrolide is associated with cross-resistance to other macrolides. Development of resistance causes particular concern in dual therapies that rely entirely on the clarithromycin component for antimicrobial effect. Unlike metronidazole-resistant strains in which the metronidazole-containing regimens still have reasonable cure rates, clarithromycin-resistant strains are rarely eliminated with clarithromycin-containing regimens. Response rates are 0% to 25%.[50]

Amoxicillin and tetracycline resistance have both been described but apparently are still rare. *H pylori* in general rapidly develops resistance to many antibiotics (eg, quinolones).[50]

Effect of Resistance on Outcome of Therapy

If *H pylori* is truly resistant to an antibiotic, administration of that antibiotic will have no effect, and treatment will fail. As noted previously, the local concentration of orally administered antibiotics is very high; thus, in vitro resistance may not equal in vivo resistance. Achieving reasonable resistance expectations should be possible by examining the outcome of trials in which two of the three agents of a triple therapy are given. We need to know the results of any therapy in the presence of sensitive and resistant *H pylori*. Such detailed data are largely unavailable or consist of very small samples, widening the 95% confidence intervals and making it difficult to judge the actual rate of success (eg, fair or very poor).

Table 5: Effect of Resistance to an Agent on Success of Antimicrobial Therapy

Therapy: Combination metronidazole, proton pump inhibitor, and clarithromycin

Resistant to	Success
None	98%
Metronidazole	70%
Clarithromycin	10%
Both	0%

Table 5 lists our estimates of the efficacy of the widely used metronidazole/PPI/clarithromycin triple therapy and shows the effect of resistance to one agent. These estimates are based on our experience and data from the literature. Loss of metronidazole leaves the PPI plus clarithromycin; we expect to achieve a cure rate of about 70%, and experience shows that we do. In contrast, clarithromycin resistance leaves only metronidazole/PPI dual therapy, which has a much inferior outcome. As we obtain more data, we will understand whether we can predict outcome based on the known cure rates of the remaining drugs, or if a component provides synergy. Synergy is most likely seen with bismuth.

Prevention of Resistance

Development of antibiotic resistance may be related in part to the *inoculum effect*, which describes a significant increase in the MIC of an antibiotic that occurs when a large number of organisms are inoculated. If the rate of development of resistance were 1 in 10 million and 100 million organisms were present (10^8), resistant *H pylori* would already be present before the antimicrobial was administered. Therefore, resistance is partly a statistical problem. Resistance may already be present at a low level and thus not develop, but is uncovered because killing the sensitive strains leaves only the preexisting population of resistant organisms. Bismuth is believed to prevent or reduce the development of resistance and may be an extremely important component of therapy. The ability of bismuth to decimate the *H pylori* population with the first dose should eliminate or diminish the inoculum effect and reduce the statistical chance of resistant strains remaining. The same reasoning can be applied to multidrug therapies.

Another potentially important phenomenon is the biofilm phenomenon: organisms attached to a surface display a significantly increased MIC toward antimicrobials. The biofilm phenomenon has been demonstrated with *H pylori* using tissue culture, and although we do not know whether this phenomenon is present in vivo, there is no reason to believe it is not.

H pylori resides 'outside' the body like gingival and skin bacteria. A form of topical therapy in the stomach is possible because the relatively small intragastric volume makes it possible to deliver a high concentration of antimicrobial agents directly to the site of infection. Fasting intragastric volume is typically less than 50 mL and rarely exceeds 500 mL postprandially, allowing small doses of antimicrobial to produce high MICs.[45] Although an isolate may show resistance to 16 mg/L of metronidazole, administration of 500 mg would expose the bacterium to concentrations as high as 1,000 mg/L and might 'overcome' the resistance as assessed in vitro. Thus, while resistance may be declared based on in vitro assessments of very low doses of antibiotics, the organism may be confronted with a bactericidal level in vivo. Better understanding of the effect of antibiotics in the gastric environment is needed, but this is difficult to study realistically. Multidrug therapy to prevent resistance is required.

Choice of Therapy After Repeated Treatment Failures (Salvage Therapy)

Treatment failure implies antibiotic resistance or failure to take the medication. The ideal approach is to culture the organism and pick a new therapy based on the result of sensitivity testing. The best salvage therapies are based on BMT triple therapy and consist of quadruple therapy or replacing the metronidazole with another drug. The bismuth-containing quadruple therapy is the best salvage treatment in the absence of pretreatment antibiotic susceptibility. Replacing metronidazole with furazolidone (100 mg three times daily) is an alternative. There are data indicating that high-dose amoxicillin-omeprazole therapy is also effective. The doses are amoxicillin 1 g and omeprazole 40 mg given three times a day for 14 days. The success rate is probably about 75%. Because esomeprazole and omeprazole are essentially equivalent, it is likely that esomeprazole can replace omeprazole, but this has not been examined clinically. It seems obvious that if this high-dose dual therapy is reasonably effective, it might be improved by the addition of another drug. We recommend a fluoroquinolone once daily (levofloxacin 500 mg, moxifloxacin 400 mg, or gatifloxacin 400 mg), or rifabutin 150 mg twice daily.[51,52] We prefer a fluoroquinolone, assuming one had not been previously used.

Future Approaches to Antimicrobial Therapy

Overall, the data are consistent with higher doses and longer durations of antibiotics and PPIs[53] giving the best results. Improved therapies for *H pylori* are clearly needed. Unfortunately, the pharmaceutical industry has little incentive for sponsoring new trials because it cannot obtain exclusivity for drugs that are generally off-patent, and the duration of therapy is short. In our opinion, the most promising therapy is called *sequential therapy*.[54,55] The approach is to first suppress the vast majority of the resident *H pylori* population with drugs that are rarely associated with resistance. Then, when few *H pylori* remain, a third or third and fourth drug are added to 'clean up.' This approach has been a basis for the use of bismuth.[56] Recent sequential therapies have involved amoxicillin and a PPI for 5 days followed by clarithromycin and metronidazole.[56] Recently, it has been shown that this approach is superior to the same combination (PPI, clarithromycin, amoxicillin) given in the traditional manner.[55] We are currently testing a combination of high-dose PPI (eg, omeprazole 40 mg t.i.d.) and amoxicillin (1 g t.i.d.) for 5 days followed by a fluoroquinolone (eg, gatifloxacin 400 mg once daily or metronidazole 500 mg t.i.d.) for an additional 7 days.

Therapy is likely to be only temporarily effective in developing countries where high rates of reinfection are the rule.[57,58] The low likelihood of rapid improvements in sanitation and standards of living in these areas makes development of a vaccine a high priority.[59,60]

What to Tell the Patient

Poor compliance is the controllable factor most likely to result in treatment failure. A motivated patient therefore is a key to success. Patients should be instructed in what they can expect, doses, durations, possible side effects, and the necessity of completing the entire course of therapy (ie, not stopping when they feel better). Patients who use tobacco should be educated about the benefits of stopping. Clear written instructions about when and how to take the pills are helpful. Patients receiving a bismuth-containing compound should be told to expect a black discoloration to their stools. The most prominent side effect of clarithromycin is a metallic taste, and many patients find this bothersome; forewarning is important. Gastric distress from the drugs can be reduced by instructing the patient to take them with food. Pharmacists may routinely label tetracycline as not to be taken with food. We administer all drugs with food because this greatly simplifies the treatment regimen and is not associated with a reduction in cure rates. This approach requires education of the patient and the pharmacist that *H pylori* is an infection in the stomach, and the rules of thumb derived from measurements of blood levels may not apply. As noted above, food tends to retain the drug longer in the stomach and distribute it throughout the stomach.

The patient should understand that *H pylori* infection damages the stomach and that cure of the infection will result in healing of the damage and likely cure peptic ulcer disease. This discussion is particularly important for nonulcer dyspepsia patients. These patients should be told the benefits of therapy but that their symptoms may not be directly related to the infection and thus may not resolve.

Many ulcer patients have accepted the prevailing myths concerning ulcer disease, and it helps to directly address these usually unspoken concerns. For example, many patients believe the myths that stress caused their condition and that a special diet or milk is important in treatment.

Whom to Treat

The groups of patients with *H pylori* infection for whom treatment is recommended continue to increase. All patients with gastric or duodenal ulcers who are *H pylori* positive should receive antibiotic therapy, whether they present with an initial ulcer or a recurrence. Patients on maintenance antiulcer therapy who have *H pylori* infection should receive anti-*H pylori* therapy. Research initially focused on resolution of the patient's symptoms. Current considerations about the desirability of treating an infectious disease include the expected outcomes of the disease, whether the infection can be successfully treated, and the risks of not treating the infection in relationship to the uninfected population. Asymptomatic *H pylori* infection provides a reservoir for transmission of disease to the uninfected community. The risks of asymptomatic *H pylori* infection are not trivial and exceed those of asymptomatic tuberculosis and syphilis.[61,62] The concept that *H pylori* infection is trivial except in a small proportion of patients is no longer tenable. The question is now best stated as "for whom can we deny therapy for *H pylori* infection?" We believe that clinicians cannot deny treatment once diagnosis has been established. The question is therefore not whom to treat but whom to test (Figure 2), because evidence of infection, with few exceptions, demands treatment.

Until an effective vaccine or a simple effective therapy with limited or mild side effects is available, the question of whom to test is best considered a public health problem. The benefits of therapy are clear, but we are constrained by cost, the existence of drug-resistant *H pylori*, and the impracticality of treating half the population.

Is Pretreatment Testing Always Required?

We believe that patients should not receive antibiotic therapy if they do not have an infection because they can achieve no benefit. Researchers have suggested that because *H pylori* is so common in patients with duodenal ulcer disease, this population may be an exception, and confirmation of the infection may be optional. We do not agree, because duodenal ulcer patients who have ulcers attributable to non-*Helicobacter* etiologies derive only the risks associated with antibiotic therapy, with a delay in obtaining the correct diagnosis (eg, Zollinger-Ellison syndrome). The widespread availability of noninvasive testing (eg, serologic tests, urea breath tests [UBTs], stool antigen testing) has made pretreatment testing mandatory. We have a low threshold for diagnosis and treatment and would test and treat those at increased risk for peptic ulcer or gastric cancer. Such individuals can be identified with some certainty based on the presence of disease in a first-degree relative. The bottom line is that no one deserves, needs, wants, or benefits from *H pylori* infection.

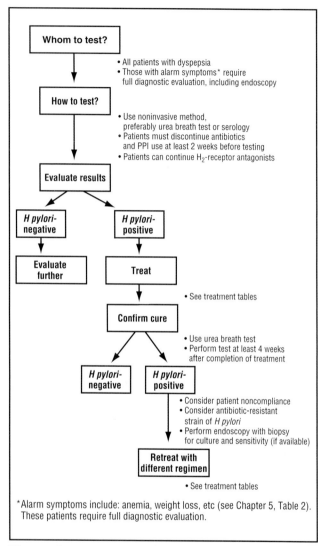

Figure 2: Management algorithm for dyspeptic patients without alarm symptoms.

Assessment of the Results of Therapy

While few disagree that it is important to confirm the presence of infection before instituting antibiotic therapy, the role of post-therapy testing remained controversial until noninvasive tests became widely available. The UBT and the stool antigen test make noninvasive testing simple and affordable. The need for post-therapy confirmation is related to the likelihood of poor outcome with continued infection coupled with the fact that the overall clinical effectiveness of current therapies is on the order of 60% to 85%. Testing is especially important for patients with a history of ulcer complications, severe symptomatic peptic ulcer disease, or gastric mucosa-associated lymphoid tissue (MALT) lymphoma. Ulcer complications are expected in approximately 2% a year of those with ulcer disease, and in 10% to 12% a year of those with a recent ulcer complication. Failure to cure the infection in a patient with peptic ulcer is associated with return of symptoms, recurrent ulcer disease, continuing risk of development of ulcer complications, need for more tests, and additional treatment for peptic ulcer. Patients with nonulcer dyspepsia and asymptomatic family members of a patient with gastric cancer or duodenal ulcer retain their original risks of developing a serious manifestation of *H pylori* infection. They remain a reservoir for transmission of the infection to others in the environment, especially family members. Post-therapy testing is now the standard of care; failure to recommend and offer post-therapy testing is reasonable grounds for malpractice litigation if the ulcer recurs and an ulcer complication ensues.

Recurrence of symptoms should always prompt retesting before retreatment, because many with recurrent symptoms will have symptoms unrelated to *H pylori* infection. For example, many conditions will respond temporarily to antibiotics (eg, small bowel bacterial overgrowth), and it is imprudent to attempt a second course of therapy unless the clinician is confident that the infection is still present.

Options for Assessing Success of Therapy

A noninvasive and inexpensive UBT or stool antigen test is sufficient. Whichever test is used, it is important to wait a sufficient time after the course of antibiotics to ensure that residual *H pylori* have multiplied to detectable levels. The data suggest that a 4-week hiatus is preferable for histology, culture, or UBT. Six to 8 weeks is required if one uses the stool antigen test. PPIs should be stopped at least 1 week before testing because, as noted previously, PPIs have a weak antimicrobial effect and lead to false-negative test results for all tests that require actively growing *H pylori* (eg, UBT, stool antigen testing, culture, rapid urease testing, histology). Because it evaluates the entire stomach, the UBT is the first to return to positive in the case of treatment failure. One week of stoppage of PPIs may be sufficient, but 2 weeks is preferred. Because H_2-receptor antagonists have no effect on *H pylori*, they can be continued up to the day before testing. In contrast, researchers have suggested that PPIs and H_2-receptor antagonists adversely affect the ^{14}C breath test and should be stopped several days to 1 week before using that test.[63] Stopping antisecretory therapy can be difficult for some patients, and antisecretory therapy should not be discontinued for patients with complicated ulcers until the clinician confirms that the infection has been eliminated. All patients should be admonished against taking bismuth-containing products or antibiotics during the month before testing.

Is It Necessary to Wait 4 Weeks After Therapy Before Testing for Confirmation of Cure?

As noted previously, although the UBT becomes positive soon after therapy is discontinued, the duration of suppression of the infection varies, thus the recommendation to wait at least 4 weeks before performing the UBT or 6 to 8 weeks if using stool antigen testing. Some have attempted to focus on when a positive stool antigen test can be interpreted as failure instead of on how many extra tests might be needed to be confident that a negative test actually reflected cure. For example, in a recent study, it was found that false-positive stool antigen tests were present 3 days after ending antibiotic therapy. In contrast, there were no false-positive tests at 7 days, but approximately one half of those whose infection had been cured had false-negative tests.[64] Even at 35 days post-therapy, the false-positive rate remained 6% (95% CI = 0.2% to 28.7%), which is consistent with the suggestion that it is preferable to wait 6 to 8 weeks after therapy before confirmation of cure with the stool antigen test.[65] With culture, histology, rapid urease testing, or the UBT, a positive test any time after the end of therapy is indicative of treatment failure. However, a negative test is difficult to interpret before that time because prolonged suppression, rather than cure, may be present. If confidence that the infection is cured is critical, endoscopy with biopsy could be performed or the previously negative test can be repeated 8 or 12 weeks post-therapy.

Ideally, if the patient has undergone multiple courses of antibiotics for *H pylori* and remains infected, cultures with susceptibility testing should be performed. Confirmation of cure at endoscopy requires at least three and preferably four gastric mucosal biopsies (see Chapter 5). Large-cup biopsies are preferred, two from the antrum and one or two from the corpus. The rapid urease test can also be done, but, if the indication for follow-up is previously complicated ulcer disease, histologic evaluation may be the better choice, and regardless of the outcome, the mucosal biopsy specimens should be sent for histologic examination by an experienced pathologist.

Serologic testing is not useful for confirming the outcome of therapy. While a statistically significant fall in antibody titer after therapy can readily be detected in a population of patients, physicians are not interested in the statistics of large groups, but rather want data about the outcome of therapy in an individual patient. Serologic tests have very low specificity and sensitivity for detection of cure in an individual patient because antibody levels remain elevated for a long time (eg, 'serologic scar'). A negative test correlates with cure, but is unusual before 2 years after therapy. Recurrent infection is associated with a return of test positivity.

Strategies to Prevent Ulcer Recurrence

Long-term or 'maintenance' antisecretory medication was once the mainstay of therapy for ulcers but has been replaced by antibiotic therapy directed against *H pylori*. However, antisecretory therapy still has a role in selected circumstances. As noted previously, patients with a history of ulcer complications, such as bleeding, should continue antisecretory therapy until cure of the infection is confirmed.[16] Maintenance antisecretory therapy for an additional 2 to 4 weeks after the antibiotic therapy to ensure healing is also indicated for those with severe symptoms or with active ulcers. Patients with resistant *H pylori* who fail therapy can be given antisecretory therapy to prevent ulcer recurrence and reduce complications. We can still rely on data from the pre-*H pylori* era about the efficacy of this form of therapy while awaiting new therapies. Elderly patients with comorbid disease and peptic ulcer, or others with short life expectancy in whom antibiotic therapy may be considered too complicated or otherwise unwise, should receive long-term or 'lifetime' antisecretory therapy instead of anti-*H pylori* therapy.

Economics of Therapy

The cost of acid-related disorders is substantial, in direct medical expenditures for therapy and in time lost from work. Data from Kaiser Permanente estimated the total annual excess costs to the HMO of acid-related disorders at $60 million. Patients with peptic ulcer disease had the highest annual costs of the acid-related disorders group, with approximately $2,000 in costs during the first 6 months after diagnosis.[66] Of the entire US population, researchers estimate that almost 5 million people have peptic ulcer disease, with roughly 29 million days of diminished work activity per year.[67] Also, 3 million physician visits are directly related to symptoms of ulcer disease.

Because of the significant costs of acid-related disease, several investigations have studied the cost-effectiveness of treating *H pylori*. At the outset, it seems obvious that if 1 or 2 weeks of therapy could cure a chronic, often lifelong disease, it would be cheaper than lifelong therapy, no matter how inexpensive the therapy. As expected, cure of *H pylori* infection has repeatedly been shown to be cost-effective. Most studies involved modeling. For example, when 727 patients with active duodenal ulcers were followed for 15 years, the expected costs per patient of the chosen therapy using a Markov chain model were $995 for antibiotic combination therapy, $10,350 for intermittent antisecretory therapy, $11,186 for maintenance antisecretory therapy, and $17,661 for a highly selective vagotomy.[68]

One study used a medical practice model over a 12-month period.[67] This study showed that immediate treatment of *H pylori* was less expensive than a short course of antisecretory therapy followed by treatment of the infection only after the first ulcer recurrence. Cure of the infection was also less expensive than long-term maintenance antisecretory therapy. The initial approach with noninvasive methods is less expensive than endoscopy in cost, safety, and efficacy.

Several studies have investigated the cost-effectiveness of treating *H pylori* in nonulcer dyspepsia patients. Ofman et al used a decision analysis and showed that initial *H pylori* eradication therapy was most cost-effective.[69] However, several important preconditions included a history and physical examination to exclude those with serious organic disease, narrowing the included patients to only those with nonulcer dyspepsia. Also, follow-up was mandated 4 to 8 weeks after eradication therapy; those with persistent symptoms underwent endoscopy at that point. Patients who presented with new nonulcer dyspepsia and were found to have *H pylori* underwent eradication combination therapy. During 6-month follow-up, those patients in whom the infection had been treated had a reduced need for invasive studies compared with those without *H pylori* who did not undergo eradication therapy.[66]

Cost-effective modeling studies do not account for many variables, such as time lost from work, poor quality of life of the patient with ulcer disease, the effect of the disease on the family, the risk of ulcer complications, development of cancer, and transmission of the disease to family members. We need to practice cost-effective and evidence-based medicine. The evidence is that *H pylori* infection is a serious disease. Charges that are easily measured often differ from true costs or best patient care. We believe that no one needs, wants, or deserves an *H pylori* infection. The ultimate goal should be to eliminate it from mankind as we eliminated smallpox.

References

1.   Graham DY: Evolution of concepts regarding *Helicobacter pylori*: from a cause of gastritis to a public health problem. *Am J Gastroenterol* 1994;89:469-472.

2.   Marshall BJ: The use of bismuth in gastroenterology. The ACG Committee on FDA-Related Matters. American College of Gastroenterology. *Am J Gastroenterol* 1991;86:16-25.

3.   Graham DY, Evans DG: Prevention of diarrhea caused by enterotoxigenic *Escherichia coli*: lessons learned with volunteers. *Rev Infect Dis* 1990;12:S68-S72.

4.   Blecker U, Gold BD: Treatment of *Helicobacter pylori* infection: a review. *Pediatr Infect Dis J* 1997;16:391-399.

5.   Graham DY, Lew GM, Evans DG Jr, et al: Effect of triple therapy (antibiotics plus bismuth) on duodenal ulcer healing. A randomized controlled trial. *Ann Intern Med* 1991;115:266-269.

6.   Miehlke S, Graham DY: Antimicrobial therapy of peptic ulcer. *Int J Antimicrob Agents* 1997;8:171-178.

7.   Graham DY: Clarithromycin for treatment of *Helicobacter pylori* infections. *Eur J Gastroenterol Hepatol* 1995;7:S55-S58.

8.   Liu WZ, Xiao SD, Shi Y, et al: Furazolidone-containing short-term triple therapies are effective in the treatment of *Helicobacter pylori* infection. *Aliment Pharmacol Ther* 1999;13:317-322.

9.   Segura AM, Gutierrez O, Otero W, et al: Furazolidone, amox-icillin, bismuth triple therapy for *Helicobacter pylori* infection. *Aliment Pharmacol Ther* 1997;11:529-532.

10.   Leung WK, Graham DY: Rescue therapy for *Helicobacter pylori*. *Curr Treat Options Gastroenterol* 2002;5:133-138.

11.   Shiotani A, Nurgalieva ZZ, Yamaoka Y, et al: *Helicobacter pylori*. *Med Clin North Am* 2000;84:1125-1136.

12.   Gisbert JP, Calvet X, Bujanda L, et al: 'Rescue' therapy with rifabutin after multiple *Helicobacter pylori* treatment failures. *Helicobacter* 2003;8:90-94.

13.   Moore RA, Beckthold B, Wong S, et al: Nucleotide sequence of the gyrA gene and characterization of ciprofloxacin-resistant mutants of *Helicobacter pylori*. *Antimicrob Agents Chemother* 1995;39:107-111.

14.   Tankovic J, Lascols C, Sculo Q, et al: Single and double mu-tations in gyrA but not in gyrB are associated with low- and high-level fluoroquinolone resistance in *Helicobacter pylori*. *Antimicrob Agents Chemother* 2003;47:3942-3944.

15.   Nakajima S, Graham DY, Hattori T, et al: Strategy for treat-ment of *Helicobacter pylori* infection in adults, II. Practical policy in 2000. *Curr Pharm Des* 2000;6:1515-1529.

16.   Miehlke S, Bayerdorffer E, Graham DY: Treatment of *Helicobacter pylori* infection. *Semin Gastrointest Dis* 2001;12:167-179.

17.   Graham DY: A reliable cure for *Helicobacter pylori* infec-tion? *Gut* 1995;37:154-156.

18.   Borody TJ, Cole P, Noonan S, et al: Recurrence of duodenal ulcer and *Campylobacter pylori* infection after eradication. *Med J Aust* 1989;151:431-435.

19.   Graham DY: Determinants of antimicrobial effectiveness in *H pylori* gastritis. In: Hunt RH, Tytgat GN, eds. *Helicobacter py-lori*: *Basic Mechanisms to Clinical Cure*. Dordrecht, Netherlands, Kluwer Academic Publishers, 1994, pp 531-537.

20. Chiba N, Rao BV, Rademaker JW, et al: Meta-analysis of the efficacy of antibiotic therapy in eradicating *Helicobacter pylori*. *Am J Gastroenterol* 1992;87:1716-1727.

21. Dore MP, Leandro G, Realdi G, et al: Effect of pretreatment antibiotic resistance to metronidazole and clarithromycin on outcome of *Helicobacter pylori* therapy: a meta-analytical approach. *Dig Dis Sci* 2000;45:68-76.

22. Gisbert JP, Khorrami S, Calvet X, et al: Meta-analysis: proton pump inhibitors vs. H_2-receptor antagonists—their efficacy with antibiotics in *Helicobacter pylori* eradication. *Aliment Pharmacol Ther* 2003;18:757-766.

23. Laheij RJ, Rossum LG, Jansen JB, et al: Evaluation of treatment regimens to cure *Helicobacter pylori* infection–a meta-analysis. *Aliment Pharmacol Ther* 1999;13:857-864.

24. Broutet N, Tchamgoue S, Pereira E, et al: Risk factors for failure of *Helicobacter pylori* therapy—results of an individual data analysis of 2751 patients. *Aliment Pharmacol Ther* 2003;17:99-109.

25. Fischbach LA, Goodman KJ, Feldman M, et al: Sources of variation of *Helicobacter pylori* treatment success in adults worldwide: a meta-analysis. *Int J Epidemiol* 2002;31:128-139.

26. Moayyedi P, Feltbower R, Crocombe W, et al: The effectiveness of omeprazole, clarithromycin and tinidazole in eradicating *Helicobacter pylori* in a community screen and treat programme. Leeds Help Study Group. *Aliment Pharmacol Ther* 2000;14:719-728.

27. Gisbert JP, Khorrami S, Calvet X, et al: Systematic review: Rabeprazole-based therapies in *Helicobacter pylori* eradication. *Aliment Pharmacol Ther* 2003;17:751-764.

28. Boixeda D, Martin De Argila C, Bermejo F, et al: Seven-day proton pump inhibitor, amoxicillin and clarithromycin triple therapy. Factors that influence *Helicobacter pylori* eradications success. *Rev Esp Enferm Dig* 2003;95:206-209, 202-205.

29. Ellenrieder V, Fensterer H, Waurick M, et al: Influence of clarithromycin dosage on pantoprazole combined triple therapy for eradication of *Helicobacter pylori*. *Aliment Pharmacol Ther* 1998;12:613-618.

30. Huang J, Hunt RH: The importance of clarithromycin dose in the management of *Helicobacter pylori* infection: a meta-analysis of triple therapies with a proton pump inhibitor, clarithromycin

and amoxicillin or metronidazole. *Aliment Pharmacol Ther* 1999;13:719-729.

31. Gold BD, Colletti RB, Abbott M, et al: *Helicobacter pylori* infection in children: recommendations for diagnosis and treatment. *J Pediatr Gastroenterol Nutr* 2000;31:490-497.

32. Vergara M, Vallve M, Gisbert JP, et al: Meta-analysis: comparative efficacy of different proton-pump inhibitors in triple therapy for *Helicobacter pylori* eradication. *Aliment Pharmacol Ther* 2003;18:647-654.

33. Graham DY, Hammoud F, El-Zimaity HM, et al: Meta-analysis: proton pump inhibitor or H_2-receptor antagonist for *Helicobacter pylori* eradication. *Aliment Pharmacol Ther* 2003;17:1229-1236.

34. Miwa H, Nagahara A, Kurosawa A, et al: Is antimicrobial susceptibility testing necessary before second-line treatment for *Helicobacter pylori* infection? *Aliment Pharmacol Ther* 2003;17:1545-1551.

35. McMahon BJ, Hennessy TW, Bensler JM, et al: The relationship among previous antimicrobial use, antimicrobial resistance, and treatment outcomes for *Helicobacter pylori* infections. *Ann Intern Med* 2003;139:463-469.

36. Megraud F, Lamouliatte H: Review article: the treatment of refractory *Helicobacter pylori* infection. *Aliment Pharmacol Ther* 2003;17:1333-1343.

37. Graham DY: Therapy of *Helicobacter pylori*: current status and issues. *Gastroenterology* 2000;118:S2-S8.

38. van der Wouden EJ, Thijs JC, van Zwet AA, et al: The influence of in vitro nitroimidazole resistance on the efficacy of nitroimidazole-containing anti-*Helicobacter pylori* regimens: a meta-analysis. *Am J Gastroenterol* 1999;94:1751-1759.

39. Graham DY, Osato MS, Hoffman J, et al: Metronidazole containing quadruple therapy for infection with metronidazole resistant *Helicobacter pylori*: a prospective study. *Aliment Pharmacol Ther* 2000;14:745-750.

40. Graham DY, Dore MP: The QUADRATE study: a proposal for a change in the reporting of pharmaceutical supported trials. *Gastroenterology* 2003;125:639.

41. Yousfi MM, el-Zimaity HM, Cole RA, et al: Metronidazole, ranitidine and clarithromycin combination for treatment of

Helicobacter pylori infection (modified Bazzoli's triple therapy). *Aliment Pharmacol Ther* 1996;10:119-122.

42. Lazzaroni M, Bargiggia S, Porro GB: Triple therapy with ranitidine or lansoprazole in the treatment of *Helicobacter pylori*-associated duodenal ulcer. *Am J Gastroenterol* 1997;92:649-652.

43. van der Hulst RW, Keller JJ, Rauws EA, et al: Treatment of *Helicobacter pylori* infection in humans: a review of the world literature. *Helicobacter* 1996;1:6-19.

44. de Boer WA, Driessen WM, Jansz AR, et al: Quadruple therapy compared with dual therapy for eradication of *Helicobacter pylori* in ulcer patients: results of a randomized prospective single-centre study. *Eur J Gastroenterol Hepatol* 1995;7:1189-1194.

45. Graham DY, Borsch GM: The who's and when's of therapy for *Helicobacter pylori*. *Am J Gastroenterol* 1990;85:1552-1555.

46. Grant R, Grossman MI, Ivy AC: Histological changes in the gastric mucosa during digestion and their relationship to mucosal growth. *Gastroenterology* 1953;25:218-231.

47. Willems G: Trophicity of gastric epithelium and its regulation. In: Mignon M, Galmiche JP, eds. *Safe and Effective Control of Acid Secretion*. Paris, John Libbey Eurotext, 1988, pp 39-50.

48. Graham DY: Variability in the outcome of treatment of *Helicobacter pylori* infection: a critical analysis. In: Hunt RH, Tytgat GN, eds. *Helicobacter pylori: Basic Mechanisms to Clinical Cure 1998*. Dordrecht, Netherlands, Kluwer Academic Publishers, 1998.

49. Walt RP: Metronidazole-resistant *H pylori*—of questionable clinical importance. *Lancet* 1996;348:489-490.

50. Graham DY, de Boer WA, Tytgat GN: Choosing the best anti-*Helicobacter pylori* therapy: effect of antimicrobial resistance. *Am J Gastroenterol* 1996;91:1072-1076.

51. Nista EC, Candelli M, Cremonini F, et al: Levofloxacin-based triple therapy vs. quadruple therapy in second-line *Helicobacter pylori* treatment: a randomized trial. *Aliment Pharmacol Ther* 2003;18:627-633.

52. Wong WM, Gu Q, Lam SK, et al: Randomized controlled study of rabeprazole, levofloxacin and rifabutin triple therapy vs. quadruple therapy as second-line treatment for *Helicobacter pylori* infection. *Aliment Pharmacol Ther* 2003;17:553-560.

53. Vallve M, Vergara M, Gisbert JP, et al: Single vs. double dose of a proton pump inhibitor in triple therapy for *Helicobacter py-*

lori eradication: a meta-analysis. *Aliment Pharmacol Ther* 2002;16:1149-1156.

54.   Hassan C, De Francesco V, Zullo A, et al: Sequential treatment for *Helicobacter pylori* eradication in duodenal ulcer patients: improving the cost of pharmacotherapy. *Aliment Pharmacol Ther* 2003;18:641-646.

55.   Zullo A, Vaira D, Vakil N, et al: High eradication rates of *Helicobacter pylori* with a new sequential treatment. *Aliment Pharmacol Ther* 2003;17:719-726.

56.   Graham DY: Antibiotic resistance in *Helicobacter pylori*: implications for therapy. *Gastroenterology* 1998;115:1272-1277.

57.   Soto G, Bautista CT, Roth DE, et al: *Helicobacter pylori* re-infection is common in Peruvian adults after antibiotic eradication therapy. *J Infect Dis* 2003;188:1263-1275.

58.   Leal-Herrera Y, Torres J, Monath TP, et al: High rates of recurrence and of transient reinfections of *Helicobacter pylori* in a population with high prevalence of infection. *Am J Gastroenterol* 2003;98:2395-2402.

59.   Frenck RW Jr, Clemens J: Helicobacter in the developing world. *Microbes Infect* 2003;5:705-713.

60.   Ruggiero P, Peppoloni S, Rappuoli R, et al: The quest for a vaccine against *Helicobacter pylori*: how to move from mouse to man? *Microbes Infect* 2003;5:749-756.

61.   Axon A, Forman D: *Helicobacter* gastroduodenitis: a serious infectious disease. *BMJ* 1997;314:1430-1431.

62.   Graham DY: Can therapy ever be denied for *Helicobacter pylori* infection? *Gastroenterology* 1997;113:S113-S117.

63.   Chey WD, Woods M, Scheiman JM, et al: Lansoprazole and ranitidine affect the accuracy of the ^{14}C-urea breath test by a pH-dependent mechanism. *Am J Gastroenterol* 1997;92:446-450.

64.   Vaire D, Vakil N, Menegatti M, et al: The stool antigen test for detection of *Helicobacter pylori* after eradication therapy. *Ann Intern Med* 2002;136:280-287.

65.   Graham DY, Qureshi WA: Markers of infection. In: Mobley HL, Mendz GL, Hazell SL (eds). *Helicobacter pylori: Physiology and Genetics.* Washington, DC, ASM Press, 2001, pp 499-510.

66.   Jones R, Tait C, Sladen G, et al: A trial of a test-and-treat strategy for *Helicobacter pylori* positive dyspeptic patients in general practice. *Int J Clin Pract* 1999;53:413-416.

67. Vakil N, Fennerty B: The economics of eradicating *Helicobacter pylori* infection in duodenal ulcer disease. *Am J Med* 1996;100:60S-63S.

68. Sonnenberg A, Townsend WF: Costs of duodenal ulcer therapy with antibiotics. *Arch Intern Med* 1995;155:922-928.

69. Ofman JJ, Etchason J, Fullerton S, et al: Management strategies for *Helicobacter pylori*-seropositive patients with dyspepsia: clinical and economic consequences. *Ann Intern Med* 1997; 126:280-291.

Chapter **7**

Helicobacter pylori, Gastroesophageal Reflux Disease, Barrett's Esophagus, and Adenocarcinoma of the Distal Esophagus

Two issues regarding *Helicobacter pylori* infection and gastroesophageal reflux disease (GERD) have caused unnecessary confusion among practicing physicians and opinion leaders, especially nongastroenterologists, and have led to some patients being denied appropriate therapy. The first is whether patients with GERD should be evaluated for *H pylori* infection. The other is whether treatment of *H pylori* will somehow trigger GERD in those without it.

GERD

Many patients have significant gastroesophageal reflux without disease. Disease requires abnormalities in the barrier that normally prevents reflux of gastric contents into the esophagus, and gastric contents with sufficient toxicity (eg, acidity) to cause pain, mucosal damage, or both. In patients with intact stomachs, acid and pepsin in the gastric contents are responsible for the esophageal damage. Successful therapies for GERD have focused on antisecretory drugs and have become increasingly successful as therapy has changed from antacids through H_2-receptor antagonists to proton pump inhibitors (PPIs). Thus, increasingly potent antisecretory therapies have led to increasingly effective clinical responses. *H pylori* infection could theoretically be involved in GERD by affecting either the antireflux barrier or gastric acid secretion.[1] *H pylori* has little or no effect on the antireflux barrier but, depending on the pattern and severity of gastritis, can have predictable effects on acid secretion.

Esophageal Acid Load

One key to understanding GERD is the concept of esophageal acid load. The severity of GERD and the presence of associated complications (eg, peptic stricture, Barrett's esophagus, adenocarcinoma of the upper stomach and lower esophagus) are related to acid exposure. The esophageal acid load is an expression of the acidity and the length of time that acid is in contact with the esophageal mucosa (eg, acidity times duration). A patient can be in one of two groups regarding esophageal reflux: those with trivial esophageal acid loads, and those with sufficient esophageal acid loads to, under the proper circumstances, develop disease. The presence of gastroesophageal reflux per se does not equate with the presence of clinical GERD. *Disease* implies the presence of symptoms or mucosal damage, and it is possible to have a large amount of reflux with neither, provided the esophageal acid load remains below the threshold that causes damage. The goal of current potent antisecretory therapy is to reduce the esophageal acid load below that critical threshold.

Figure 1 shows the relationship between acidity and time of exposure to the severity of GERD. In the plot on the right, the amount of acid secretion is held constant and the reflux time is varied. In this scenario, the esophageal acid load is directly related to the duration of reflux, and the severity of the GERD increases directly in rela-

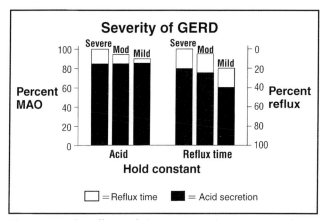

Figure 1: The effects of changing acid secretion and percent reflux time (esophageal acid load) on the severity of gastroesophageal reflux disease (GERD). Acid secretion is represented as percent of pentagastrin-stimulated maximal acid output (MAO), and reflux as the proportion of time that gastric contents reflux into the esophagus. The data are presented as a concept model showing that the severity of gastroesophageal reflux is related to the esophageal acid load whether dominated by the amount of acid secretion or the amount of reflux time.

tion to the increase in the duration of the reflux. The left plot shows the effect of keeping reflux time constant and varying the degree of acid secretion. Here, the severity of GERD is directly related to acid secretion, and it should be obvious that even a modest change in acid secretion can have a major effect on the outcome of a patient with GERD or on a patient with reflux but without disease.

Helicobacter pylori and Corpus Gastritis

Cure of *H pylori* infection can increase or decrease the esophageal acid load, depending on the pattern and sever-

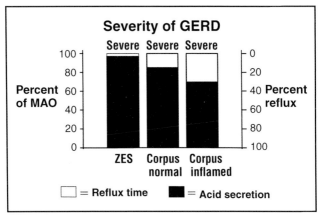

Figure 2: This plot illustrates that the same outcome (eg, severe esophagitis) can occur with markedly different patterns of acid secretion and with different patterns of gastritis, ranging from none to moderate corpus gastritis. For any patient, there will be thresholds for development of gastroesophageal reflux disease (GERD) and for different severities of GERD among those with reflux. MAO = maximal acid output, ZES = Zollinger-Ellison syndrome.

ity of gastritis. Cure of the infection will have little or no effect on the reflux barrier and will not cause GERD to occur among those without preexisting gastroesophageal reflux (eg, those with reflux but without disease). Just as cure of *H pylori* has predictable effects on the pattern and severity of gastritis, so do the pattern and severity of gastritis have predictable effects on acid secretion, the important determinant of esophageal acid load (Figure 2). It is evident that a patient with high, sustained acid secretion (eg, a patient with the Zollinger-Ellison syndrome) might develop GERD with a modest degree of reflux. In contrast, a patient with normal acid secretion would require a longer reflux time, and a patient with reduced acid secretion would require a very large acid exposure to exceed the GERD threshold.

Effect of Antisecretory Therapy on *Helicobacter pylori* Gastritis

The use of antisecretory drugs in patients with active *H pylori* infection also has predictable effects on the pattern and severity of gastritis because antisecretory drugs are associated with a worsening of the severity of corpus gastritis.[1] Decades ago, it was recognized that gastritis tended to remain restricted to the antrum in patients with duodenal ulcer but that it rapidly extended into the gastric corpus when acid secretion was reduced, for example, by selective parietal cell vagotomy. Acid or acid secretion seemed to be the factor that limited the rate of progression of gastritis from the antrum into the corpus. We suggested that acid was also the factor that was responsible for inhibiting *H pylori* from interacting with the corpus mucosa in duodenal ulcer patients.[2] Subsequent experiments showed that antisecretory therapy of any kind seemed to remove or reduce this restriction, allowing an *H pylori*-corpus mucosal interaction, and was associated with rapid worsening of corpus gastritis, reminiscent of the accelerated progression of gastritis seen after acid-reducing surgery. It was suggested that because the rapid worsening of corpus gastritis tended to produce a pattern of gastritis associated with gastric cancer, acid suppression therapy might ultimately be harmful by increasing the risk of developing gastric cancer.[3,4] These findings led the most recent Maastricht Consensus conference to recommend *H pylori* eradication for all patients in whom long-term antisecretory drug therapy is contemplated.[5]

Cure of *Helicobacter pylori* Among Patients With Clinical GERD

By definition, patients with GERD have a sufficiently high esophageal acid load to cause disease. Thus, few will have preexisting significant corpus gastritis, which by itself, would reduce acid secretion (see below). Cure of the *H pylori* infection restores the normal down-regulation of acid secretion associated with gastric distention or antral acidification and reduces the duration of acid secretion in response to a meal.[6] Cure of *H pylori* should therefore reduce the esophageal acid load. This change in regulation of acid secretion is not associated with more than a slight reduction in the stomach's ability to secrete acid in response to pentagastrin. Thus, in most patients, one would expect no change in GERD symptoms or in antisecretory drug requirement following cure of an *H pylori* infection. A small to modest proportion of patients would be expected to improve, with reflux symptoms becoming either subclinical or requiring less intensive therapy, and this is what has been typically observed in clinical practice.[7] Such improvement is likely limited to patients whose esophageal acid load was just above threshold and then fell below.

One potential effect of anti-*H pylori* therapy is that PPI therapy, which is less effective in suppressing acid at night among *H pylori*-negative patients compared to those with *H pylori* gastritis, decreases in effectiveness after cure of an *H pylori* infection. Further studies showed that this effect was related to the small amount of ammonia produced by the hydrolysis of urea by *H pylori* urease, which was sufficient in the unstimulated state to neutralize the small amount of acid made by newly formed or previously uninhibited acid pumps on parietal cells.[8] Hydrogen ion concentration is a log scale. A pH of 1 equals 100 mmol/L acid, and a pH of 4 is achieved at a concentration of 0.1 mmol/L of acid. The pH in the stomach can rise above 4 with PPI therapy as the small amount of acid made is neutralized by the ammonia produced, but it will often fall below 4 if no *H pylori* are present to produce the ammonia. In contrast to PPIs, an evening dose of an H_2-receptor antagonist demonstrated effectiveness in maintaining the intragastric pH at 4 or higher.[9] Investigators interested in

GERD subsequently used intraesophageal pH measurements that assessed the pH in the stomach indirectly, and confirmed the observation that PPIs were less effective than H_2-receptor antagonists after *H pylori* eradication or among those with no *H pylori* infection. They named this previously described phenomenon *acid breakthrough*.[10] It is now widely recognized that a combination of a PPI in the morning and an H_2-receptor antagonist at night generally provides better acid control than does twice-a-day PPI therapy, and this may be the preferred approach for those with GERD and no *H pylori* infection or after *H pylori* eradication.

Helicobacter pylori Among Patients Without Clinical GERD

Epidemiologic studies suggest a possible inverse relationship between *H pylori* and GERD.[1] For example, prospective endoscopic studies among dyspeptic patients in regions where gastric carcinoma is common (eg, Korea) show a very low prevalence of erosive GERD. In contrast, in regions where gastric cancer is rare (eg, United States), a high proportion of dyspeptic patients have GERD. In both populations, the extent and severity of corpus inflammation dictate the range of acid secretion and therefore the esophageal acid load among that proportion of the population that has significant gastroesophageal reflux. It follows that the average acid secretion is higher in a population without *H pylori* infection (thus lacking *H pylori*-associated corpus gastritis and decreased acid secretion) than in a population with *H pylori* infection, which will have individuals with decreased acid secretion because of corpus gastritis.

We hypothesize that the extent and prevalence of gastroesophageal barrier dysfunction are similar among different populations, but the prevalence of GERD is not. Acid secretion is lowest among populations or groups with severe corpus gastritis. Thus, the incidence of GERD is expected to be inversely related to the incidence of gastric

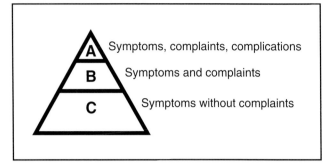

Figure 3: The pyramid or 'iceberg' represents the populations of patients with gastroesophageal reflux. The largest group are those with mild disease who self-medicate with over-the-counter drugs and rarely, if ever, visit doctors because of their symptoms. The smallest group consists of those who visit gastroenterologists because of severe disease requiring continuous high-dose therapy. Adapted from Graham DY: Therapeutic efficacy revisited. *Dig Dis Sci* 1984;29:589-590.

cancer: if the incidence of gastric cancer falls, the incidence of GERD will increase. In the early 1980s, we suggested that the population of GERD patients should be thought of as a pyramid or iceberg with three groups, the largest being subclinical (symptoms without complaints)[11,12] (Figure 3). This iceberg analogy subsequently has been widely adapted by others.[13] We now propose that there is a fourth group, those with gastroesophageal reflux without disease (Figure 4), characterized as having an esophageal acid load below the threshold for causing symptoms or damage. In countries where atrophic pangastritis (and gastric cancer) are common, most patients with gastroesophageal reflux will fall within this group. The reciprocal changes that have occurred in the epidemiology of *H pylori*-related diseases, duodenal ulcer and gastric cancer, have been accompanied

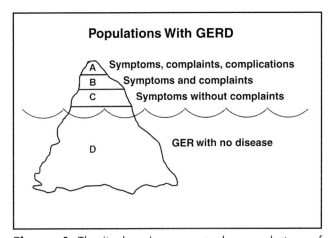

Figure 4: The 'iceberg' represents the populations of patients with gastroesophageal reflux (GER) in countries where chronic atrophic gastritis and gastric cancer are common and gastroesophageal reflux disease (GERD) is rare. In such areas, the *Helicobacter pylori* gastritis-associated reductions in acid secretion are such that patients have neither symptoms nor endoscopic changes despite the presence of gastroesophageal reflux. This is shown as a group unrecognized in the West (group D).

or preceded by changes in the average pattern of gastritis. As the rate of acquisition of atrophic pangastritis fell and the average ability to secrete acid rose, the incidence of gastric cancer declined, and the incidence of duodenal ulcer increased. Because GERD depends on the esophageal acid load, its prevalence tended to follow that of duodenal ulcer. We expect the incidence of gastroesophageal reflux without disease will decrease in Japan and Korea as they move toward a pattern similar to that found in the United States (ie, a Westernization of the pattern of upper gastrointestinal diseases).

GERD Appearing
After *Helicobacter pylori* Eradication

We noted in the late 1980s that the epidemiology of adenocarcinoma of the esophagus, a known complication of GERD, appeared to be changing, particularly increasing in white men, the same group in whom *H pylori* infection was disappearing. We postulated that the two events were related such that the loss of *H pylori* resulted in an increase in the average acid secretion and thus in the severity of GERD and the incidence of complications among those with GERD.[1] Other investigators, while accepting the association between the two diseases, carried the association further and proposed that *H pylori* was actually 'protective', postulating that there may be a beneficial effect of *H pylori* infection.[14] We believe that the apparent controversy is the result of misunderstandings about the role of *H pylori* in the pathogenesis of gastroesophageal reflux and the relationship of gastroesophageal reflux to GERD.[1,4,15] The presence of gastroesophageal reflux is a function of the effectiveness of the barrier mechanisms at the esophagogastric junction preventing reflux. The effectiveness of this barrier is in turn influenced by anatomic features (presence of hiatal hernia, body mass index) and by drugs and foods that impair lower esophageal function. GERD is related to the esophageal acid load, which may be affected by *H pylori* infection.[1,4,15]

GERD Among Duodenal Ulcer Patients

In the pre-*H pylori* era, it was widely recognized that duodenal ulcer disease was commonly accompanied by GERD.[16] In fact, GERD was known to become a clinical problem after peptic ulcer disease surgery in 30% to 60% of cases.[17-24] In retrospect, one should have expected GERD to appear in a similar proportion of patients with duodenal ulcer after *H pylori* eradication. Probably the most instructive report in the pre-*H pylori* era was by Casula and Jordan, who asked whether they could prevent the expected incidence of GERD among patients with duodenal ulcer undergoing highly selective vagotomy.[17] They evaluated 38 patients with duodenal ulcer and found gastroesophageal reflux in 37%. Those patients were then selected to undergo the combination of an antireflux procedure and a highly selective vagotomy, whereas those with duodenal ulcer without reflux had only a highly selective vagotomy. This approach prevented GERD from developing postsurgery among those who had surgical therapy for their duodenal ulcer disease. That gastroesophageal reflux was common among duodenal ulcer patients is not surprising, because patients with duodenal ulcer tend to have high acid secretion such that even a modest impairment of the reflux barrier is sufficient to produce an esophageal acid load of sufficient magnitude to cause GERD.

In duodenal ulcer patients, GERD may appear or worsen independent of *H pylori* as antisecretory therapy for duodenal ulcer is decreased or eliminated. Cure of *H pylori* is invariably associated with attempts to eliminate chronic antisecretory therapy; therefore, cure of *H pylori* infection in a patient with duodenal ulcer would be expected to increase the severity of GERD because regular use of antisecretory drugs would no longer be necessary to treat the symptoms of duodenal ulcer, and thus the average esophageal acid load would increase in that antisecretory therapy was no longer taken regularly.

GERD in Corpus Gastritis

Decades ago, it was also recognized that corpus gastritis was associated with a reduction in acid secretion out of proportion to the decrease in the number of parietal cells. Several studies have tested the hypothesis that cure of *H pylori* infection among those with corpus gastritis will increase acid output.[25] It is now recognized that cure of the infection removes the inflammation-associated inhibition of parietal cell function among those with corpus

Table 1: Acid Load After Cure of _H pylori_

	H pylori⁺	Cured
Time pH <4	60 min	60 min
Average pH	3.5	2.2
H^+ (mEq/L)	0.55	8.25
Acid load (H^+ x time)	33.0	495.0
Load	1x	15x

gastritis and, depending on the severity of inflammation and the number of parietal cells, can produce marked increases in gastric acidity. In countries where gastric cancer is common, corpus gastritis is common, acid secretion is low, and clinical GERD is uncommon. Cure of _H pylori_ infection in patients with corpus gastritis will increase their acid secretion and, thus, the esophageal acid load among those with reflux. Esophageal acid load is sensitive to acid concentration. The changes in esophageal acid load can be systematically overlooked with the current techniques used to assess intraesophageal pH. For example, acid reflux is somewhat arbitrarily defined as intraesophageal pH lower than 4. By definition, gastroesophageal reflux of gastric contents with a pH greater than 4 cannot be identified. It is interesting that one can still measure the presence of gastroesophageal reflux by identifying the presence of bilirubin in the esophagus or by the new impedence technique. The traditional approach, to use episodes of intraesophageal pH below 4 to define reflux, allows major changes in esophageal acid load to remain unrecognized. For example, consider a hypothetical situation of two patients who both reflux 60 minutes per day. In neither patient does the reflux time change following _H pylori_ eradication. One patient has severe corpus gastritis and loss of parietal cells with an intragastric pH of 4.1 before therapy, decreasing to 3.9 after cure of the infection. That patient would be scored as having developed reflux as a consequence of therapy, but, because the esophageal acid would be trivial, gastroesophageal reflux would not be expected to manifest as GERD. The second patient has less severe corpus gastritis. Pretherapy, the intragastric pH was 3.5 (0.55 mmol/L), falling to 2.2 post-therapy (8.25 mmol/L). Cure of the infection would be associated with an increase in acid load (concentration x time) of 15-fold (from 33 mmol/h H^+ to 495 mmol/h H^+), and yet the pH reflux test would be interpreted as 'no change' because the time that the pH was below 4 had not changed (Table 1). This hypothetical situation shows how a modest change in acidity can result in a major increase in esophageal acid load, and one that would be unrecognized using modern approaches to assess the severity of GERD. It also follows that GERD will only occur among the population of patients with pretherapy gastroesophageal reflux in whom the esophageal acid load increased above threshold. 'Protection' is related to the extent and severity of corpus gastritis.

Role of Cytokine-Associated Gene A (cagA)

Epidemiologic evidence has shown that infection with *H pylori* with a functional *cag* pathogenicity island is associated with an increased risk of peptic ulcer and gastric cancer. There are also data that infection with these strains is associated with a reduced risk of GERD and its complication, adenocarcinoma of the distal esophagus.[1] The mechanism is related to the fact that an intact *cag* pathogenicity island is associated with enhanced mucosal IL-8 secretion and more severe gastritis. The general concept that CagA-positive *H pylori* might be beneficial with regard to GERD and esophageal adenocarcinoma is flawed because duodenal ulcer is associated with CagA-positive

H pylori, antral-predominant gastritis, high acid secretion, and, among those with gastroesophageal reflux, GERD. CagA-positive *H pylori* infection is also associated with corpus gastritis, low acid secretion, and gastric ulcer and gastric cancer. Those with gastroesophageal reflux are protected from GERD by the low esophageal acid load. Thus, it is corpus gastritis with low acid secretion that actually protects against GERD and its complications, such as Barrett's esophagus and adenocarcinoma of the esophagus and gastric cardia. A CagA-positive *H pylori* infection will only offer protection if it acts as a biologic antisecretory agent by reducing acid secretion in those with reflux.[1] Therefore 'protection' is restricted to a small subgroup of patients. The group with CagA-positive *H pylori* and antral-predominant gastritis continues to experience a risk for development of duodenal ulcer of approximately 1% per year and is also at high risk (depending on the barrier function) of developing GERD. Those with the best protection (ie, those with gastroesophageal reflux and atrophic pangastritis) have a risk of gastric cancer of approximately 1% per year (See Figure 9, Chapter 4). The incidence of adenocarcinoma of the distal esophagus among the highest-risk group (white men) is much less than 6 per 100,000 per year, which contrasts markedly with the risk for gastric cancer among those with atrophic pangastritis, which is in the range of 1,000 per 100,000 per year. This risk of gastric cancer also extends to those at low risk of adenocarcinoma of the esophagus, such as women, blacks, and most of the population without gastroesophageal reflux who are 'immune' from Barrett's esophagus independent of the presence or absence of *H pylori* infection.

Conclusions

In the last century, Western populations with *H pylori* infection experienced a change in the pattern of gastritis, primarily a reduction in the rate of corpus gastritis. These effects were likely primarily caused by changes in diet associated with the year-round availability of fresh fruits and vegetables.[26] This resulted in a change in the epidemiology of *H pylori*-related diseases where diseases that were common, such as atrophic gastritis, gastric ulcer, and gastric cancer, were replaced by duodenal ulcer. The prevalence of *H pylori* infection also declined as changes in sanitation led to a fall in the rate of acquisition of *H pylori* infections. Generally, this led to better health in the population. Nonetheless, one group, those with gastroesophageal reflux, experienced an increase in the esophageal acid load leading to increases in incidence of GERD and adenocarcinoma of the distal esophagus. The fall in incidence of corpus gastritis led to an increase in acid secretion and thus virtual disappearance of the group of patients with gastroesophageal reflux without symptoms or disease (Figure 5). This process is now occurring in countries where gastric cancer is still common and GERD is rare. We predict that the incidence of GERD in these countries (where GERD is now rare) will become similar to that seen in Western populations coincident with the improvements in gastric histology and acid secretion. The proposal not to treat all *H pylori* infections as 'bad' begs the question about who is at risk for this cancer and therefore who might be 'protected'. White men are at highest risk, more specifically, white men with gastroesophageal reflux. In the United States, the prevalence of *H pylori* in white men is now less than 15%. Therefore, any increase in incidence of adenocarcinoma related to loss of *H pylori* has already occurred, and any additional increase in prevalence will be related to aging of the population (as adenocarcinoma of the distal esophagus is typically a disease of the elderly). Whether cure of the *H pylori* infection increases acid production depends on the pattern of gastritis. The more severe the corpus inflammation, the more acid secretion is depressed and the more it will increase post-therapy. As one would

Figure 5: This illustration depicts the change in the presentation of gastroesophageal reflux associated with the change in the average pattern of gastritis from an atrophic pangastritis to a nonatrophic gastritis or normal stomach. Gastric cancer became rare while duodenal ulcer and gastroesophageal reflux disease (GERD) became problems among the populations with *Helicobacter pylori* infection. Thus, the prevalence of GERD is inversely related to that of gastric cancer. This change in patterns occurred during the period from the middle of the 19th century to the later part of the 20th century and is now occurring in many countries.

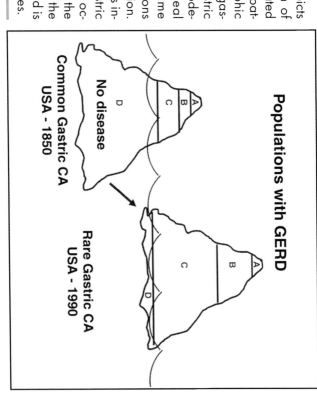

predict, infection with CagA-positive *H pylori* that causes the highest degree of inflammation will be the most 'protective'.[1] The patient with *H pylori*-related 'protection' against GERD can be characterized as a patient with gastroesophageal reflux and severe corpus gastritis (CagA-positive *H pylori*) such that the esophageal acid load remains below the threshold for esophageal disease. That pattern of gastritis also identifies patients at highest risk for gastric ulcer and for gastric cancer. The absence of *H pylori* infection in a population results in duodenal ulcer, gastric ulcer, and gastric cancer becoming rare diseases. Until recently, adenocarcinoma of the distal esophagus was an extremely rare disease. It is still very rare, and despite the dramatic increase in incidence, will likely remain rare. In contrast, in 1930, gastric cancer was the most common cancer worldwide, and while the world celebrates the dramatic decline in incidence, in nonwhite men in the United States, the incidence is still greater than 20 per 100,000 (Figure 6). There should be no controversy about whether *H pylori* is protective against anything because it is not, and it should be eradicated whenever and wherever it is discovered.

The increase in the incidence of adenocarcinoma of the distal esophagus has been used by others to suggest that elimination of *H pylori* from society may lead to an epidemic of new problems. However, all beneficial actions are associated with new problems. For example, increased life span increased the occurrence of cancer, heart disease, stroke, and other diseases of aging. Barrett's esophagus and adenocarcinoma of the gastroesophageal junction exist in developing countries, despite the almost universal prevalence of *H pylori* infection. They exist in those with antral-predominant gastritis, and they are increasing in the United States as the frequency of *H pylori*-associated atrophic gastritis has decreased more rapidly than *H pylori* infection, probably because of changes in diet. Even though esophageal junction cancer is the most rapidly increasing

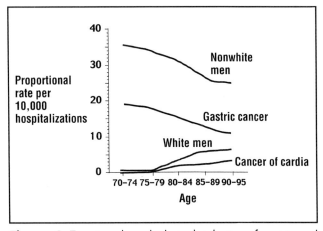

Figure 6: Time trends and ethnic distribution of gastric and esophageal adenocarcinoma. This figure shows that while gastric cancer in whites has become a rare disease coincident with the loss of *Helicobacter pylori* from the population, there has been an increase in adenocarcinoma of the esophagus. Nonetheless, the increase has changed what was a very rare disease into a rare one. The use of percent increase as a measure of importance provides a misleading impression of the relative importance of the change in incidence of this cancer. Adapted from El-Serag HB, Sonnenberg A: Ethnic variations in the occurrence of gastroesophageal cancers. *J Clin Gastroenterol* 1999;28:135-139.

gastrointestinal cancer, we must recognize that 'rapidly increasing' is misleading.[27] These cancers are rare and will remain so. The incidence will increase as the prevalence of antral predominant *H pylori* increases and as *H pylori* naturally disappears. *H pylori* is an unsafe biologic antisecretory agent with high morbidity. In contrast, GERD can be controlled by surgery or safe and potent antisecretory drugs, when necessary.

References

1. Graham DY, Yamaoka Y: *H pylori* and cagA: relationships with gastric cancer, duodenal ulcer, and reflux esophagitis and its complications. *Helicobacter* 1998;3:145-151.

2. Graham DY: *Campylobacter pylori* and peptic ulcer disease. *Gastroenterology* 1989;96 (suppl):615-625.

3. Kuipers EJ, Lundell L, Klinkenberg-Knol EC, et al: Atrophic gastritis and *Helicobacter pylori* infection in patients with reflux esophagitis treated with omeprazole or fundoplication. *N Engl J Med* 1996;334:1018-1022.

4. Shiotani A, Nurgalieva ZZ, Yamaoka Y, et al: *Helicobacter pylori*. *Med Clin N Am* 2000;84:1125-1136.

5. Malfertheiner P, Megraud F, O'Morain C, et al: Current concepts in the management of *Helicobacter pylori* infection—the Maastricht 2-2000 consensus report. *Aliment Pharmacol Ther* 2002; 16:167-180.

6. Dore MP, Graham DY: Pathogenesis of duodenal ulcer disease: the rest of the story. *Baillieres Best Pract Res Clin Gastroenterol* 2000;14:97-107.

7. McColl KE, Dickson A, El-Nujumi A, et al: Symptomatic benefit 1-3 years after *H. pylori* eradication in ulcer patients: impact of gastroesophageal reflux disease. *Am J Gastroenterol* 2000;95:101-105.

8. Bercík P, Verdú EF, Armstrong D, et al: The effect of ammonia on omeprazole-induced reduction of gastric acidity in subjects with *Helicobacter pylori* infection. *Am J Gastroenterol* 2000;95:947-955.

9. Labenz J, Tillenburg B, Peitz U, et al: Effect of curing *Helicobacter pylori* infection on intragastric acidity during treatment with ranitidine in patients with duodenal ulcer. *Gut* 1997;41:33-36.

10. Katz PO, Anderson C, Khoury R, et al: Gastroesophageal reflux associated with nocturnal gastric acid breakthrough on proton pump inhibitors. *Aliment Pharmacol Ther* 1998;12:1231-1234.

11. Graham DY: Therapeutic efficacy revisited. *Dig Dis Sci* 1984; 29:589-590.

12. Graham DY: Categories of patients with gastroesophageal reflux. *Arch Intern Med* 1991;151:2476.

13. Kitchin LI, Castell DO: Rationale and efficacy of conservative therapy for gastroesophageal reflux disease. *Arch Intern Med* 1991; 151:448-454.

14. Blaser MJ: Hypothesis: the changing relationships of *Helicobacter pylori* and humans: implications for health and disease. *J Infect Dis* 1999;179:1523-1530.

15. Anand BS, Graham DY: Ulcer and gastritis. *Endoscopy* 1999;31:215-225.

16. Graham DY, Dixon MF: Acid secretion, *Helicobacter pylori* infection, and peptic ulcer disease. In: Graham DY, Genta RM, Dixon MF, eds. *Gastritis.* Philadelphia, Lippincott Williams & Wilkins, 1999, pp 177-188.

17. Casula G, Jordan PH Jr: Is an antireflux procedure necessary in conjunction with parietal cell vagotomy in the absence of preoperative reflux? *Am J Surg* 1987;153:215-220.

18. Cruze K, Byron FX, Hill JT: The association of peptic ulcers and asymptomatic hiatal hernia. *Surgery* 1959;46:664-668.

19. Csendes A, Oster M, Moller JT, et al: Gastroesophageal reflux in duodenal ulcer patients before and after vagotomy. *Ann Surg* 1978;188:804-808.

20. Goldman MS Jr, Rasch JR, Wiltsie DS, et al: The incidence of esophagitis in peptic ulcer disease. *Am J Dig Dis* 1967;12:994-999.

21. Katz PO, Anderson C, Khoury R, et al: Gastro-oesophageal reflux associated with nocturnal gastric acid breakthrough on proton pump inhibitors. *Aliment Pharmacol Ther* 1998;12:1231-1234.

22. de Moraes-Filho JP, Zaterka S, Pinotti HW, et al: Esophagitis and duodenal ulcer. *Digestion* 1974;11:338-346.

23. Peghini PL, Katz PO, Bracy NA, et al: Nocturnal recovery of gastric acid secretion with twice-daily dosing of proton pump inhibitors. *Am J Gastroenterol* 1998;93:763-767.

24. Winkelstein A: Peptic esophagitis with duodenal ulcer. *Am J Surg* 1957;93:234-237.

25. Gutierrez O, Melo M, Segura AM, et al: Cure of *Helicobacter pylori* infection improves gastric acid secretion in patients with corpus gastritis. *Scand J Gastroenterol* 1997;32:664-668.

26. Graham DY: *Helicobacter pylori* infection in the pathogenesis of duodenal ulcer and gastric cancer: a model. *Gastroenterology* 1997;113:1983-1991.

27. El-Serag HB, Sonnenberg A: Ethnic variations in the occurrence of gastroesophageal cancers. *J Clin Gastroenterol* 1999;28:135-139.

Chapter 8

Pediatrics

Although infection with *Helicobacter pylori* is now recognized to be typically acquired during childhood,[1-3] the natural history of infection in childhood remains poorly understood. Data indicate that the infection frequently is acquired and lost in childhood.[4] However, whether this clearance is related to the use of antibiotics for other common infections (such as otitis media), is the natural history of the infection, or both remains unclear.[4] Some evidence suggests that reinfection is common among those aged 5 years or younger. In conditions where acquisition of the infection is common (eg, unsanitary conditions, crowding), reinfection may occur throughout childhood. The infection is most commonly acquired in childhood or when one has young children in the family.

Adults generally carry the *H pylori* they acquired as children, and the clinical manifestations of infection, such as peptic ulcer disease and gastric cancer, are actually long-term outcomes of the childhood infection. Adult acquisition of the infection is rare, with rates lower than 0.5% per year and currently lower than the rate of loss of the infection in developed countries.[5] Recently, increasing attention has been directed at understanding the role of *H pylori* in pediatrics.

Epidemiology in Childhood

In developed Western nations such as the United States, Canada, and Western Europe, few children are acquiring the infection; 3.5% of French children are infected by age 10.[3,6] The *H pylori* prevalence in Japanese children is 5% to 6%.[7]

The overall prevalence of *H pylori* infection in children in developed countries is roughly 10%, but lower socioeconomic status children may have prevalence rates of up to 30% to 40%.[5,8] Cross-sectional studies suggest that children are typically infected when they are younger than 5 years.[8]

These low rates in the first 10 years of life in children from developed countries contrast with the much higher rates in developing countries. For example, in Nigeria and Gambia, roughly half the children younger than 10 years are infected, with similarly high numbers in Algeria (45%) and the Ivory Coast (55%).[9,10] In many developing countries, prevalence rates by age 10 years are closer to 80%.[5,8]

A serologic study of American children and adolescents conducted as part of the third National Health and Nutrition Examination Survey (NHANES III, covering the years 1988-1994) evaluated 2,581 US children aged 6 to 19 years and found a seroprevalence of antibodies to *H pylori* of 24.8%.[11] The prevalence in non-Hispanic whites was 17%, compared with 40% of non-Hispanic blacks and 42% of Mexican Americans. The data on childhood prevalence rates of infection with *H pylori* from the United States are remarkably consistent.[12-16] Socioeconomic status, not ethnicity, seems to be the main risk factor associated with childhood acquisition of *H pylori*.[17]

In adults, the increase in prevalence of infection with age is thought to be a cohort effect, with higher rates seen in people born in the early years of the 20th century and decreasing rates over the subsequent years. This cohort effect reflects the different (improving) hygienic standards prevalent during childhood over the course of the last century.[18] In children, the studies support progressive acquisition of the infection. Risk factors associated with higher prevalence rates of the infection include low socioeconomic status, crowding and high-density living situations, inadequate sanitation practices, and close person-to-person contact.[16-19] Protective factors include good nutritional status; especially protective is frequent consumption of fruits, vegetables, and vitamin C.[9] Breast-feeding has also been shown to be protective.[16]

H pylori probably obtains access to the stomach by many different routes. Direct oral-oral transmission seems unlikely, whereas gastro-oral and fecal-oral transmission are good possibilities.[20,21] The only proven source is iatrogenic from *H pylori*-contaminated endoscopes or pH probes.[22,23] The results of examining *H pylori* strains obtained from family members have yielded conflicting information. Some studies have shown that the isolates are identical or very similar, supporting person-to-person transmission within the family unit or from a common source. Studies showing higher prevalence rates in institutionalized children and adults support person-to-person transmission.[18] Other studies of strains present in family members have shown the strains to be markedly different. Infection from an environmental source is likely in developing countries, and although rare, infection from an animal source cannot be entirely ruled out.[19] Molecular epidemiologic techniques allow *H pylori* to be distinguished with regard to region of origin (eg, Asia, Iberian peninsula). Studies of *H pylori* obtained within ethnic groups where marriage outside the group is infrequent have shown that strains tend to circulate within the ethnic group. For example, Hispanic individuals in the United States tend to have strains that can be traced back to Spain, those with Northern European ancestry have Northern European strains, etc.[24] These findings are consistent with the idea that the levels of household and general hygiene are the common denominators associated with transmission of the infection.

Helicobacter pylori Gastritis in Children

The association between antral gastritis and *H pylori* infection in children was confirmed soon after the initial report by Warren and Marshall, which was based on adult patients. *H pylori* infection was not found in cases of secondary gastritis, but it was present in most cases of children with primary gastritis. This implicates *H pylori* as the etiologic agent in chronic antral gastritis in children and adults.[3,4,25]

Because children rarely ingest alcohol, use tobacco, or regularly use nonsteroidal anti-inflammatory drugs (NSAIDs), the potential confounders in the association between infection with *H pylori* and gastrointestinal symptoms are fewer, making it easier to draw a correlation between infection and symptoms. Most infected children who have gastritis are asymptomatic.[5,25] Fiedorek et al[26] studied 245 healthy children who were considered asymptomatic by their parents and found that 30% were infected.[26] In contrast, cure of *H pylori* infection leads to cure of *H pylori*-related peptic ulcer in children and adults.[5,27]

Peptic Ulcer Disease

Children infected with *H pylori* develop chronic gastritis, but few progress to frank peptic ulcer disease.[25] Large pediatric centers report five to seven cases of peptic ulcer disease a year. Gastric ulcers are exceedingly rare in the pediatric population; nearly all pediatric ulcers are found in the duodenum. Primary ulcers are rarely noted in children younger than 10 years.[3,28] These children experience recurring symptoms that become quiescent during monotherapy with H_2-receptor antagonists and relapse on withdrawal of therapy.

Most ulcers seen in children are secondary and are attributable to severe stress or medication and usually present with acute hematemesis. In infants, the first sign of ulcer disease may be intestinal perforation. The mortality from secondary ulceration is significant because of associated hemorrhage and perforation, although most affected children recover quickly without chronic ulcer-related symptoms.

Treatment of *H pylori*-infected pediatric patients with peptic ulcer disease leads to resolution of the infection and the peptic ulcer disease.[29] See later section for treatment regimens.

Gastric Ulcers

Because of the exceedingly low prevalence of gastric ulcers in children, the association between *H pylori* and ulcers in the stomach has received little attention.[30] No significant prospective studies document an association between *H pylori* in the gastric mucosa of children and subsequent gastric ulceration. Prieto et al[31] investigated 270 children who underwent endoscopy; 12 had gastric ulcers and 9 had *H pylori* infection (75% prevalence among gastric ulcer patients). Roma et al[27] retrospectively reviewed 2,550 children who underwent upper-endoscopic procedures over a 9-year period in Greece. All children who had a diagnosis of primary peptic ulcer were included in the study (52 children: 10 with gastric ulcers, 42 with duodenal ulcers; 2% of 2,550 total). No significant difference in reported symptoms was found between children with ulcers and those without ulcers. The prevalence of *H pylori* was much higher among the children with duodenal ulcers (62%) when compared to children with gastric ulcers (20%). Gastric ulcers in children tend to be secondary and, as such, are not typically chronic or recurring.

Duodenal Ulcers

H pylori infection accounts for 90% to 100% of pediatric duodenal ulcers.[9] As in adults, failure to cure the *H pylori* infection is associated with ulcer relapse, and cure of the infection leads to cure of duodenal ulcer disease.[32]

Gastric MALT Lymphoma

Primary gastric mucosa-associated lymphoid tissue (MALT) lymphoma has been reported in childhood.[33,34] For example, an *H pylori*-associated MALT lymphoma presented in a 14-year-old girl as severe cachexia and nausea. She was found to have *H pylori*-associated chronic active gastritis and a MALT lymphoma. Cure of the *H pylori* infection was followed by resolution of the MALT lymphoma without chemotherapy or surgery. The patient had no relapse at 7-year follow-up. A second case involved an 11-year-old boy with a prolonged history of abdominal complaints who was found to have *H pylori* infection and gastric non-Hodgkin's lymphoma.[33] He was treated with antibiotics and a 6-month course of chemotherapy, after which he was disease-free.

Recurrent Abdominal Pain

Recurrent abdominal pain (RAP) is common, affecting at least 10% to 15% of children aged 4 to 16 years.[35] There have been many studies investigating whether there is a causal relationship between *H pylori* infection and the presence of RAP and whether eradication of the infection leads to RAP symptom resolution. While RAP is a common condition among children, the diagnostic criteria are not clear and the symptoms that fall under the rubric of "RAP" are diverse, leading to difficulty in diagnosis and in comparing studies in the literature. Also, many of the studies usually involve populations from tertiary care centers, although most patients with RAP are cared for by their primary care physicians. Nevertheless, RAP and *H pylori* infection are not associated.[36-39]

Iron Deficiency Anemia

While infection with *H pylori* and the presence of iron deficiency anemia are uncommon in children from developed countries, a connection between the two has been proposed. A recent study from Finland showed resolution of iron deficiency anemia in several children on eradication of their infection with *H pylori*.[40] Eight children who had iron deficiency anemia but did not respond to oral iron replacement were studied. All underwent upper endoscopy and were found to have *H pylori* infection with chronic active gastritis. Four weeks after antibiotic treatment, all children were given urea breath tests (UBTs); clearance of the infection was shown in seven of eight children. Hemoglobin values were corrected after successful *H pylori* eradication.

Acute *Helicobacter pylori* in Children

There have been several papers describing acute *H pylori* gastritis in adults and children.[41-48] While there is no single presentation that characterizes new-onset *H pylori*, acute infection can be suspected when acute gastric mucosal damage is found on endoscopic examination and there are no other obvious etiologies (such as chronic nonsteroidal drug use) and when the rapid urease test from biopsy material is positive.[43] In a Texas emergency department-based study, all children aged 6 months to 12 years who presented with nonsurgical abdominal pain during a 2-month period were invited to participate.[17] Of 45 patients included in the study, 18% had positive UBT and negative serology, indicating acute infection. These children had statistically significant greater vomiting, nausea, anorexia, and abdominal pain when compared with children with negative UBT.[17]

Diagnosis of *Helicobacter pylori* Infection in Children

The diagnostic tests available for adults and children generally are not different. Researchers have expressed concern that rapid urease testing of gastric mucosal biopsy material may be less accurate in children than in adults because of the small biopsy specimens typically obtained from pediatric endoscopy, leading to correspondingly lower numbers of bacteria in the biopsy tissue fragment,[9] but this has not been our experience.[49]

UBTs are ideal for children because they are noninvasive (Figure 1). Nevertheless, the dose of urea and the test meal used in children are not yet standardized, and more work is needed before this test can be the standard for very young children or infants.[50] A recent study from Dublin suggests the use of UBT in children younger than 2 years (with direct intragastric administration of ^{13}C urea, reducing the delta $^{13}CO_2$) may be complicated by false positives from oral urease-producing organisms.[51,52] Other recent

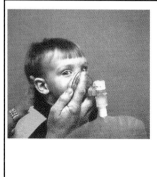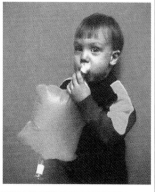

Figure 1: The ^{13}C urea breath test can be administered to children using a face mask or, if the child is old enough, by blowing into a collection bag or tube.

studies have suggested that reporting the results in terms of urea hydrolysis (eg, mg/min) effectively controls for the differences in endogenous carbon dioxide production related to age, weight, and sex. This new approach will likely allow the UBT to become the test of choice for children.

Serologic methods have been used in numerous studies involving children. *H pylori*-specific serum IgG testing is highly specific (greater than 96%) in diagnosing *H pylori* infection in children, but sensitivity is strongly age-dependent for most commercially available tests.[53] Unlike adults, in whom a positive serologic test only indicates past infection with the organism without clear indication of current status, positive serologic findings in children are more diagnostic because they have had fewer years to clear the infection. Indeed, children demonstrate a correlation between magnitude of the IgG antibodies and the bacterial load and severity of gastritis. As with adults, the precise serologic test must be chosen with care.

In the United States, the HM•CAP™ test IgG antibody to *H pylori* has proven accurate in children.[21]

Fecal tests have been developed recently for use in detecting *H pylori* infection. van Doorn et al[54] prospectively studied a stool antigen test (Premier HpSA; Meridian Diagnostics, Inc, Cincinnati, OH) in 106 children from the Netherlands. Infection was confirmed by culture and histology from gastric biopsy samples and compared with the results of stool samples obtained within 2 days of endoscopy. Sensitivity of 100% and specificity of 92% were found for the stool antigen test. Use of the stool antigen test for confirmation of infection clearance remains somewhat controversial in children,[55] and, as in adults, it is probably best to wait for approximately 8 weeks before using it to confirm *H pylori* eradication.

Saliva and urine tests have also been developed, but saliva tests currently lack the sensitivity and specificity required for clinical use. Saliva tests like the OraSure test (Epitope, Inc., Beaverton, OR), and whole blood serologic tests like FlexSure® (SmithKline Diagnostics, Palo Alto, CA), are highly specific but not very sensitive when used alone.[56] Combining salivary and systemic antibody tests improves sensitivity to levels potentially adequate for large-scale epidemiologic studies but not high enough for clinical uses.[56] We have not had any experience with the new urine tests that have been shown to be useful in adults.

Treatment

The treatment of childhood *H pylori* infection has not been extensively studied, and no consensus exists for the optimum regimen.[2,5,8] However, the benefits of treating the infection in patients with duodenal ulcer are obvious. The potential long-term benefits from treating asymptomatic children are clear, whereas the direct benefits of treating asymptomatic children while they are still children is less clear. The question is not whether to treat but when to treat, and many authorities now recommend treating all

Table 1: Treatment Studies of *H pylori* Infection in Children

First author, country	Regimen
Gottrand, France[60]	Omeprazole (Prilosec®), amoxicillin, clarithromycin (Biaxin®) 7 days; 74% clearance rate by UBT at 4 weeks post-therapy Amoxicillin, clarithromycin 7 days; 9.4% clearance rate by UBT at 4 weeks post-therapy
Shcherbakov, Russia[63]	Metronidazole (Flagyl®, Protostat®) (30-40 mg/kg/d), amoxicillin (750 mg/d), proprietary omeprazole (20-40 mg/d) for 1 week; 88.9% eradication rate Metronidazole, amoxicillin, generic omeprazole; 80% eradication rate Metronidazole, amoxicillin, ranitidine (Zantac®) (150 mg b.i.d.); 74.3% eradication rate
Oderda, Italy[57]	Lansoprazole (Prevacid®) (15 mg for children <30 kg; 30 mg for children >30 kg), amoxicillin (50 mg/kg), tinidazole (Tindamax®) (20 mg/kg) for 1 week; 73% clearance rate by UBT at 6 weeks post-therapy Placebo, amoxicillin (50 mg/kg), tinidazole (20 mg/kg) for 1 week; 65% clearance rate by UBT at 6 weeks post-therapy

UBT = urea breath test

patients, adults or children, in whom *H pylori* infection is demonstrated.[4] In children, as in adults, the concept of "do not test unless you are willing to treat" remains true.[30]

Some small-scale studies involving children have investigated various treatment options. Monotherapy is as unsuccessful in children as in adults.[29] Dual therapy yields better results but, as in adults, is not recommended. Some studies have found higher clearance rates using dual therapy in children than when the same therapy is used in adults, potentially because of lower rates of antibiotic resistance in children.[29,57] Amoxicillin and bismuth have yielded cure rates of approximately 70%.[9,58] The dual use of bismuth (4 weeks) and metronidazole (Flagyl®, Protostat®; 2 weeks) or amoxicillin and tinidazole (Tindamax®) has led to cure rates between 70% and 80%.[9,58]

Triple therapies have had greater success.[2,59-61] Walsh et al[59] in Ireland used a triple regimen of bismuth, metronidazole, and clarithromycin (Biaxin®) for a 7-day course and found a 95% eradication rate in a group of 22 infected children. Compliance was closely monitored, and the authors assert that the use of 'redi-dose' boxes (providing daily pill storage compartments with subdivisions for breakfast, lunch, dinner, and bedtime) significantly aided in patient compliance. Most experts now recommend triple therapy for 2 weeks;[2,62,63] 1-week regimens are being investigated in children but are likely to yield lower cure rates than 10- or 14-day therapies.[5,57] Furazolidone (Furoxone®) suspension is available, and this agent is probably very effective as an ingredient in combination therapy, as it is in adults. It is likely that salvage therapies using furazolidone would be successful, and we are somewhat surprised it has not been tested in primary therapy (Tables 1 and 2).

The side effects of the various regimens are similar in children and adults. Bismuth toxicity in children receiving *H pylori* therapy is not a concern. However, salicylate ingestion from the use of bismuth subsalicylate is a safety issue. For example, 30 mL of liquid Pepto-Bismol® con-

Table 2: NASPGHAN Position Statement, 2000[61]

Drug	Dosage
First-line options:	
Amoxicillin	50 mg/kg/day up to 1 g b.i.d.
Clarithromycin	15 mg/kg/day up to 500 mg b.i.d.
Omeprazole	1 mg/kg/day up to 20 mg b.i.d.; or comparable PPI
Amoxicillin	50 mg/kg/day up to 1 g b.i.d.
Metronidazole	20 mg/kg/day up to 500 mg b.i.d.
Omeprazole	1 mg/kg/day up to 20 mg b.i.d.; or comparable PPI
Clarithromycin	15 mg/kg/day up to 500 mg b.i.d.
Metronidazole	20 mg/kg/day up to 500 mg b.i.d.
Omeprazole	1 mg/kg/day up to 20 mg b.i.d.; or comparable PPI

PPI = proton pump inhibitor

tains 263 mg of salicylate. Parents should be informed of the presence of subsalicylate. Ideally, children younger than 16 years should not receive salicylate-containing compounds because of the risk of Reye's syndrome.

Suspensions are typically easier to administer to young children than tablets or pills. When suspensions are not commercially available, the capsules must be opened to create a 'homemade' suspension. This includes the proton pump inhibitors omeprazole (Prilosec®) and lansoprazole

Drug	Dosage
Second-line options:	
Bismuth subsalicylate (Pepto-Bismol®)	1 tablet (262 mg) q.i.d. or 15 mL (17.6 mg/mL q.i.d.)
Metronidazole	20 mg/kg/day up to 500 mg b.i.d.
Omeprazole	1 mg/kg/day up to 20 mg b.i.d.; or comparable PPI
+ an additional antibiotic	
Amoxicillin	50 mg/kg/day up to 1 g b.i.d.
Tetracycline	50 mg/kg/day up to 1 g b.i.d.; for children >12 years
Clarithromycin	15 mg/kg/day up to 500 mg b.i.d.
Ranitidine bismuth citrate (Tritec®, Pylorid®)	1 tablet q.i.d.
Clarithromycin	15 mg/kg/day up to 500 mg b.i.d.
Metronidazole	20 mg/kg/day up to 500 mg b.i.d.

(Prevacid®). Capsules can sometimes be opened and mixed with a small volume of an acidic liquid or food, such as apple juice, orange juice, or applesauce. However, high-pH liquids, such as milk, interfere with the granules' protective coating and should be avoided. Most of the antibiotic preparations are available as liquids, but many of these preparations, particularly those with metronidazole, are unpalatable. Mixing bad-tasting liquid medicines with grape jelly or chocolate syrup may ease administration.

Post-therapy testing to confirm eradication should be the standard of care.[4,62] It is critical to show clearance of the infection caused by the emergence and prevalence of drug-resistant strains of *H pylori*, patient noncompliance with the regimen (particularly an issue in younger children), and regimen success rates below 100% under the best of circumstances.

References

1. Deltenre M, de Koster E: How come I've got it? (A review of *Helicobacter pylori* transmission). *Eur J Gastroenterol Hepatol* 2000;12:479-482.

2. Gilger MA: Treatment of *Helicobacter pylori* infection in children. *Curr Pharm Des* 2000;6:1531-1536.

3. Torres J, Perez-Perez G, Goodman KJ, et al: A comprehensive review of the natural history of *Helicobacter pylori* infection in children. *Arch Med Res* 2000;31:431-469.

4. Malaty HM: *Helicobacter pylori* infection and eradication in paediatric patients. *Paediatr Drugs* 2000;2:357-365.

5. Rowland M, Drumm B: Clinical significance of Helicobacter infection in children. *Br Med Bull* 1998;54:95-103.

6. Blecker U: *Helicobacter pylori* disease in childhood. *Eur J Pediatr* 1996;155:753-755.

7. Kitagawa M, Natori M, Katoh M, et al: Maternal transmission of *Helicobacter pylori* in the perinatal period. *J Obstet Gynaecol Res* 2001;27:225-230.

8. Rowland M, Imrie C, Bourke B, et al: How should *Helicobacter pylori* infected children be managed? *Gut* 1999;45(Suppl 1):I36-I39.

9. Drumm B: *Helicobacter pylori* in the pediatric patient. *Gastroenterol Clin North Am* 1993;22:169-182.

10. Graham DY, Adam E, Reddy GT, et al: Seroepidemiology of *Helicobacter pylori* infection in India. Comparison of developing and developed countries. *Dig Dis Sci* 1991;36:1084-1088.

11. Staat MA, Kruszon-Moran D, McQuillan GM, et al: A population-based serologic survey of *Helicobacter pylori* infection in children and adolescents in the United States. *J Infect Dis* 1996;174:1120-1123.

12. Adler-Shohet F, Palmer P, Reed G, et al: Prevalence of *Helicobacter pylori* antibodies in normal children. *Pediatr Infect Dis J* 1996;15:172-174.

13. Fiedorek SC, Malaty HM, Evans DL, et al: Factors influencing the epidemiology of *Helicobacter pylori* infection in children. *Pediatrics* 1991;88:578-582.

14. Graham DY, Malaty HM, Evans DG, et al: Epidemiology of *Helicobacter pylori* in an asymptomatic population in the United States. Effect of age, race, and socioeconomic status. *Gastroenterology* 1991;100:1495-1501.

15. Malaty HM, Graham DY, Klein PD, et al: Transmission of *Helicobacter pylori* infection. Studies in families of healthy individuals. *Scand J Gastroenterol* 1991;26:927-932.

16. Malaty HM, Logan ND, Graham DY, et al: *Helicobacter pylori* infection in preschool and school-aged minority children: effect of socioeconomic indicators and breast-feeding practices. *Clin Infect Dis* 2001;32:1387-1392.

17. Opekun AR, Gilger MA, Denyes SM, et al: *Helicobacter pylori* infection in children of Texas. *J Pediatr Gastroenterol Nutr* 2000;31:405-410.

18. Brown LM: *Helicobacter pylori*: epidemiology and routes of transmission. *Epidemiol Rev* 2000;22:283-297.

19. Oderda G: Transmission of *Helicobacter pylori* infection. *Can J Gastroenterol* 1999;13:595-597.

20. Breuer T, Malaty HM, Graham DY: The epidemiology of *H pylori*-associated gastroduodenal diseases. In Ernst PB, Michetti P, Smith PD, eds. *The Immunobiology of H pylori: From Pathogenesis to Prevention*. Philadelphia, Lippincott-Raven, 1997, pp 1-14.

21. Chong SK, Lou Q, Asnicar MA, et al: *Helicobacter pylori* infection in recurrent abdominal pain in childhood: comparison of diagnostic tests and therapy. *Pediatrics* 1995;96:211-215.

22. Cave DR: How is *Helicobacter pylori* transmitted? *Gastroenterology* 1997;113:S9-S14.

23. Wu MS, Wang JT, Yang JC, et al: Effective reduction of *Helicobacter pylori* infection after upper gastrointestinal endoscopy by mechanical washing of the endoscope. *Hepatogastroenterology* 1996;43:1660-1664.

24. Yamaoka Y, Malaty HM, Osato MS, et al: Conservation of *Helicobacter pylori* genotypes in different ethnic groups in Houston, Texas. *J Infect Dis* 2000;181:2083-2086.

25. Imrie C, Rowland M, Bourke B, et al: Is *Helicobacter pylori* infection in childhood a risk factor for gastric cancer? *Pediatrics* 2001;107:373-380.

26.   Fiedorek SC, Casteel HB, Pumphrey CL, et al: The role of *Helicobacter pylori* in recurrent, functional abdominal pain in children. *Am J Gastroenterol* 1992;87:347-349.

27.   Roma E, Kafritsa Y, Panayiotou J, et al: Is peptic ulcer a common cause of upper gastrointestinal symptoms? *Eur J Pediatr* 2001;160:497-500.

28.   Chelimsky G, Czinn SJ: *Helicobacter pylori* infection in children: update. *Curr Opin Pediatr* 2000;12:460-462.

29.   Oderda G, Rapa A, Bona G: A systematic review of *Helicobacter pylori* eradication treatment schedules in children. *Aliment Pharmacol Ther* 2000;14(Suppl 3):59-66.

30.   Sherman P, Hassall E, Hunt RH, et al: Canadian Helicobacter Study Group Consensus Conference on the Approach to *Helicobacter pylori* Infection in Children and Adolescents. *Can J Gastroenterol* 1999;13:553-559.

31.   Prieto G, Polanco I, Larrauri J, et al: *Helicobacter pylori* infection in children: clinical, endoscopic, and histologic correlations. *J Pediatr Gastroenterol Nutr* 1992;14:420-425.

32.   Israel DM, Hassall E: Treatment and long-term follow-up of *Helicobacter pylori*-associated duodenal ulcer disease in children. *J Pediatr* 1993;123:53-58.

33.   Ashorn P, Lahde PL, Ruuska T, et al: Gastric lymphoma in an 11-year-old boy: a case report. *Med Pediatr Oncol* 1994;22:66-67.

34.   Blecker U, McKeithan TW, Hart J, et al: Resolution of *Helicobacter pylori*-associated gastric lymphoproliferative disease in a child. *Gastroenterology* 1995;109:973-977.

35.   Boyle JT: Abdominal pain. In Walker WA, Durie PR, Hamilton JR, et al, eds. *Pediatric Gastrointestinal Disease*, ed 3. Lewiston, NY, BC Decker, 2000, pp 129-149.

36.   Chen MH, Lien CH, Yang W, et al: *Helicobacter pylori* infection in recurrent abdominal pain in children—a prospective study. *Acta Paediatr Taiwan* 2001;42:278-281.

37.   Macarthur C: *Helicobacter pylori* infection and childhood recurrent abdominal pain: lack of evidence for a cause and effect relationship. *Can J Gastroenterol* 1999;13:607-610.

38.   Patwari AK: *Helicobacter pylori* infection in Indian children. *Indian J Pediatr* 1999;66:S63-S70.

39.   Wewer V, Andersen LP, Paerregaard A, et al: Treatment of *Helicobacter pylori* in children with recurrent abdominal pain. *Helicobacter* 2001;6:244-248.

40.   Ashorn M, Ruuska T, Makipernaa A: *Helicobacter pylori* and iron deficiency anaemia in children. *Scand J Gastroenterol* 2001;36:701-705.

41.   Barbosa AJ, Queiroz DM, Mendes EN, et al: *Campylobacter pylori* associated acute gastritis in a child. *J Clin Pathol* 1989; 42:779.

42.   Frommer DJ, Carrick J, Lee A, et al: Acute presentation of *Campylobacter pylori* gastritis. *Am J Gastroenterol* 1988;83:1168-1171.

43.   Graham DY: Community acquired acute *Helicobacter pylori* gastritis. *J Gastroenterol Hepatol* 2000;15:1353-1355.

44.   Mitchell JD, Mitchell HM, Tobias V: Acute *Helicobacter pylori* infection in an infant, associated with gastric ulceration and serological evidence of intra-familial transmission. *Am J Gastroenterol* 1992;87:382-386.

45.   Moriai T, Hirahara N: Clinical course of acute gastric mucosal lesions caused by acute infection with *Helicobacter pylori*. *N Engl J Med* 1999;341:456-457.

46.   Nomura H, Miyake K, Kashiwagi S, et al: A short-term eradication therapy for *Helicobacter pylori* acute gastritis. *J Gastroenterol Hepatol* 2000;15:1377-1381.

47.   Rocha GA, Queiroz DM, Mendes EN, et al: *Helicobacter pylori* acute gastritis: histological, endoscopical, clinical, and therapeutic features. *Am J Gastroenterol* 1991;86:1592-1595.

48.   Takata T, Shirotani T, Okada M, et al: Acute hemorrhagic gastropathy with multiple shallow ulcers and duodenitis caused by a laboratory infection of *Helicobacter pylori*. *Gastrointest Endosc* 1998;47:291-294.

49.   Yousfi MM, El-Zimaity HM, Cole RA, et al: Detection of *Helicobacter pylori* by rapid urease tests: is biopsy size a critical variable? *Gastrointest Endosc* 1996;43:222-224.

50.   Deslandres C: [13]C urea breath testing to diagnose *Helicobacter pylori* infection in children. *Can J Gastroenterol* 1999;13:567-570.

51.   Imrie C, Rowland M, Bourke B, et al: Limitations to carbon 13-labeled urea breath testing for *Helicobacter pylori* in infants. *J Pediatr* 2001;139:734-737.

52.   Kindermann A, Demmelmair H, Koletzko B, et al: Influence of age on 13C-urea breath test results in children. *J Pediatr Gastroenterol Nutr* 2000;30:85-91.

53. Kindermann A, Konstantopoulos N, Lehn N, et al: Evaluation of two commercial enzyme immunoassays, testing immunoglobulin G (IgG) and IgA responses, for diagnosis of *Helicobacter pylori* infection in children. *J Clin Microbiol* 2001;39:3591-3596.

54. van Doorn OJ, Bosman DK, van't Hoff BW, et al: *Helicobacter pylori* Stool Antigen test: a reliable non-invasive test for the diagnosis of *Helicobacter pylori* infection in children. *Eur J Gastroenterol Hepatol* 2001;13:1061-1065.

55. Kabir S: Detection of *Helicobacter pylori* in faeces by culture, PCR and enzyme immunoassay. *J Med Microbiol* 2001; 50:1021-1029.

56. Malaty HM, Logan ND, Graham DY, et al: *Helicobacter pylori* infection in asymptomatic children: comparison of diagnostic tests. *Helicobacter* 2000;5:155-159.

57. Oderda G, Marinello D, Lerro P, et al: Double versus triple therapy for childhood *Helicobacter pylori* gastritis: a double blind multicentre trial. *Gut* 2001;49:A77.

58. Rowland M, Drumm B: *Helicobacter pylori* infection and peptic ulcer disease in children. *Curr Opin Pediatr* 1995;7:553-559.

59. Walsh D, Goggin N, Rowland M, et al: One week treatment for *Helicobacter pylori* infection. *Arch Dis Child* 1997;76:352-355.

60. Gottrand F, Kalach N, Spyckerelle C, et al: Omeprazole combined with amoxicillin and clarithromycin in the eradication of *Helicobacter pylori* in children with gastritis: A prospective randomized double-blind trial. *J Pediatr* 2001;139:664-668.

61. Shcherbakov PL, Filin VA, Volkov IA, et al: A randomized comparison of triple therapy *Helicobacter pylori* eradication regimens in children with peptic ulcers. *J Int Med Res* 2001;29:147-153.

62. Gold BD, Colletti RB, Abbott M, et al: *Helicobacter pylori* infection in children: recommendations for diagnosis and treatment. *J Pediatr Gastroenterol Nutr* 2000;31:490-497.

63. Oderda G: Management of *Helicobacter pylori* infection in children. *Gut* 1998;43(Suppl 1):S10-S13.

Chapter 9

Future Considerations: Vaccines and Trends in Research

To meet the goal of eradicating *Helicobacter pylori* infection, new strategies must be investigated. Vaccines to prevent the infection and possibly to treat existing infections are the most promising. Active research is directed at this goal, in animal models and, recently, in human trials. An understanding of the immune response to *Helicobacter* infection helps clarify the ongoing research effort.

Immune Response Against *Helicobacter* Infection

The natural immune response induces a very strong local and serum antibody response but fails to clear the infection. Because of the chronic nature of the infection and low rate of spontaneous cure, these antibodies seem to be ineffective.[1-3] Infection leads to secretory IgA directed against the bacteria, which may help protect the stomach lining from future infection.[3] Lee et al[4] postulated that active infections can be reduced by the action of IgA: bacteria may be removed by 'immune exclusion,' whereby secretory IgA binds to urease on the surface of *H pylori*. The bacteria can become cross-linked, trapped in the mucus, and then removed from the stomach by the regular actions of peristalsis. This 'immune exclusion' mechanism has been shown with *Campylobacter jejuni*, *Salmonella typhi*, and *Vibrio cholera*.[4,5]

In addition to antibody responses to the infection, the immune system is also stimulated by various cytokines. Interleukin-8 is induced by the bacterium, which in turn attracts and activates neutrophils.[6] Such neutrophilic infiltration not only can help eradicate the infection, but also may contribute to gastric injury through release of normally intracellular enzymes. Helper cells are also involved in the immune response to the infection. *H pylori* seems to activate T_H1 helper cells, leading to increased IgG production. T_H2 cells produce a more effective immune response, which drives IgA production and assists in clearing the infection.[1-7]

Infection of mice with *Helicobacter* species results in a strong serum IgG response and a minor IgA response. Effective vaccination results in a dramatic serum and local immune response, with a correlation between protection from infection and the specific levels of secretory IgA against *H pylori* surface proteins.

Vaccines

The three components believed to be necessary for *Helicobacter* vaccines are: (a) identification of antigens that protect against infection, (b) development of an animal model that accurately reflects the results in humans, and (c) development of safe and effective mucosal adjuvants. Antigens now receiving the most attention for vaccine trials include urease, flagella proteins, adhesion molecules (required for bacterial attachment to the stomach wall), VacA, CagA, and the 60,000 molecular weight heat shock protein.[3] Urease appears to be a good choice because it constitutes more than 6% of the total soluble protein of the bacterium; it is found in the cytosol and on the surface, where it is exposed to IgA molecules; and it is constitutively expressed throughout the course of infection.[5] Current research examines mixtures of antigens because single antigens are unlikely to be effective in humans.

The gastrointestinal tract develops tolerance to orally ingested substances such that protein antigens are usually poorly immunogenic. Thus, an effective oral vaccine requires a mucosal adjuvant. Various adjuvants have been investigated for use with oral immunization trials. Cholera toxin and *Escherichia coli* heat-labile toxin (LT) are two widely used adjuvants in animal experiments, but both are too toxic for routine use in humans. One promising candidate is a detoxified mutant of LT, LTK63, which lacks toxic activity but can function as a powerful adjuvant. The active site of the enzyme has a single amino acid change. LTK63 has shown success in preliminary animal models.

Early Vaccine Success Against *Helicobacter pylori*

Much research has been directed at finding a vaccine against *Helicobacter*. Czinn and Nedrud[8,9] showed it was possible to immunize via the oral route by administering whole-cell sonicate preparations of the bacteria to mice and ferrets, which led to gastric and intestinal IgA mucosal immune responses. Experiments by Czinn, and also by Chen, later showed that mice that had previously received *Helicobacter felis* sonicates (in combination with cholera toxin adjuvant) were then protected against infection when challenged with *H felis*.[8-10] Other groups used only the urease protein in their immunization experiments, instead of whole-cell sonicates. Oral urease alone protected these mice against infection with *H felis*. These experiments were important in showing that protective antibodies could be generated against a mucosal infection that, in the natural state, rarely produces protective antibody.

Models have changed over the last several years from using the related but nonulcerogenic, nonadherent *H felis* to *H pylori* in animal models.[11] Laboratory strains of *H pylori* typically fail to infect normal rodents, which is why the original articles in the field used *Helicobacter mustelae* and *H felis* strains (for ferrets and mice, respectively). Several laboratories developed animal models using mice and a strain of *H pylori*. The Sydney strain, which produces reliable, reproducible infection in mice, has been distributed to vaccine researchers.[12]

Purified urease was used in mice experiments by Lee et al[4] using the subunits of urease (ureA and ureB) that had been cloned into an *Escherichia coli* vector. This enzyme was nonfunctional (unable to generate ammonia) because of the exclusion of an operon for nickel ion incorporation, and as little as 5 mg was found to protect mice. As expected, an adjuvant was required for induction of an IgA response, as well as for protection against challenge. Acambis (Cambridge, MA) is using a recombinant urease (rUrease) in phase I human trials.[1,13]

Therapeutic Vaccination

Oral vaccination that protects against infection is possible. Many investigators are extending the concept of vaccination to therapy for current infection. Using the *H felis* model, Doidge et al[14] infected germ-free mice with *H felis*. One month later, the animals were vaccinated with *H felis* whole-cell sonicate and cholera toxin adjuvant four times over 20 days. The animals were assessed at 1, 2, and 3 months postvaccination for evidence of infection (urease test and histology). A high proportion of mice at each assessment had cleared the infection (70% to 95%, compared with only 9% of the control group). OraVax has also demonstrated the use of vaccines as therapy using the rUrease vaccine. Mice were infected with *H felis* and then vaccinated either with rUrease and LT, or with LT adjuvant alone. Similar to the results of Doidge, 70% to 90% of the vaccinated mice cleared the infection. Recent studies in mice and beagle dogs using a parenteral vaccination with CagA, VacA, and NapA has proven successful to prevent *H pylori* infection and as therapy for active infection.[15-19] Actual cure may not occur often; rather, a marked reduction in bacterial load occurs that may be sufficient to prevent disease or to render the infection more susceptible to antimicrobial therapy.

The Future

We expect to better understand the pathophysiology of *H pylori*-related diseases, as well as better appreciate the gravity of *H pylori* infection.[20,21] Experiments designed to understand the interaction between *H pylori* and the gastric mucosa have already resulted in a much better understanding of gastric physiology. We expect this trend to continue. In addition, the new field of gastric mucosal immunology has blossomed and has provided many new insights. We expect that one outcome of the development of a vaccine against *H pylori* infection will be the ability to design and produce oral vaccines for many other mucosal pathogens.

The demonstrated ability of *H pylori* to develop resistance to antibiotics will lead to increasing antibiotic resistance. This will make current therapies less effective, as well as spur the pharmaceutical industry to develop new antibiotics. Gastric cancer, *H pylori*-related peptic ulcer, and primary gastric lymphoma will continue to decrease in prevalence and may largely become rare or historic diseases. Much work remains before this goal can be achieved.

References

1.   Kotloff KL: *Helicobacter pylori* and gastroduodenal disorders: new approaches for prevention, diagnosis and treatment. *Vaccine* 1996;14:1174-1175.

2.   Lee A, Buck F: Vaccination and mucosal responses to *Helicobacter pylori* infection. *Aliment Pharmacol Ther* 1996;10: 129-138.

3.   Telford JL, Ghiara P: Prospects for the development of a vaccine against *Helicobacter pylori. Drugs* 1996;52:799-804.

4.   Lee CK, Weltzin R, Thomas WD Jr, et al: Oral immunization with recombinant *Helicobacter pylori* urease induces secretory IgA antibodies and protects mice from challenge with *Helicobacter felis. J Infect Dis* 1995;172:161-172.

5.   Lee CK, Monath TP: Strategies for the development of effective *H pylori* vaccines. In: Ernst PB, Michetti P, Smith PD, eds.

The Immunobiology of H pylori: *From Pathogenesis to Prevention*. Philadelphia, Lippincott-Raven, 1997, pp 297-310.

6.   Crabtree JE: Virulence factors of *H pylori* and their effect on chemokine production. In: Ernst PB, Michetti P, Smith PD, eds. *The Immunobiology of* H pylori: *From Pathogenesis to Prevention*. Philadelphia, Lippincott-Raven, 1997, pp 101-112.

7.   Bamford KB, Hunt R, Muller M, et al: Gastric T cells and *H pylori*: regulation of pathogenesis and prevention. In: Ernst PB, Michetti P, Smith PD, eds. *The Immunobiology of* H pylori: *From Pathogenesis to Prevention*. Philadelphia, Lippincott-Raven, 1997, pp 213-226.

8.   Nedrud JG, Czinn SJ: Oral immunization for the prevention and treatment of infection with *Helicobacter*. In: Ernst PB, Michetti P, Smith PD, eds. *The Immunobiology of* H pylori: *From Pathogenesis to Prevention*. Philadelphia, Lippincott-Raven, 1997, pp 273-286.

9.   Czinn SJ, Nedrud JG: Oral immunization against *Helicobacter pylori*. *Infect Immun* 1991;59:2359-2363.

10.   Chen M, Lee A, Hazell S: Immunisation against gastric helicobacter infection in a mouse/*Helicobacter felis* model. *Lancet* 1992;339:1120-1121.

11.   Lee A, Fox JG: Animal models for vaccine development. In: Ernst PB, Michetti P, Smith PD, et al, eds. *The Immunobiology of* H pylori: *From Pathogenesis to Prevention*. Philadelphia, Lippincott-Raven, 1997, pp 255-272.

12.   Lee A, O'Rourke J, De Ungria MC, et al: A standardized mouse model of *Helicobacter pylori* infection: introducing the Sydney strain. *Gastroenterology* 1997;112:1386-1397.

13.   Kreiss C, Buclin T, Cosma M, et al: Safety of oral immunisation with recombinant urease in patients with *Helicobacter pylori* infection. *Lancet* 1996;347:1630-1631.

14.   Doidge C, Crust I, Lee A, et al: Therapeutic immunisation against *Helicobacter* infection. *Lancet* 1994;343:914-915.

15.   Del Giudice G, Ghiara P, Rappuoli R: Experimental model of *Helicobacter pylori* infection. *Ital J Gastroenterol Hepatol* 1998;30(Suppl 3):S261-S263.

16.   Del Giudice G, Covacci A, Telford JL, et al: The design of vaccines against *Helicobacter pylori* and their development. *Annu Rev Immunol* 2001;19:523-563.

17.   Ghiara P, Rossi M, Marchetti M, et al: Therapeutic intragastric vaccination against *Helicobacter pylori* in mice eradicates an otherwise chronic infection and confers protection against reinfection. *Infect Immun* 1997;65:4996-5002.

18.   Rossi G, Rossi M, Vitali CG, et al: A conventional beagle dog model for acute and chronic infection with *Helicobacter pylori*. *Infect Immun* 1999;67:3112-3120.

19.   Satin B, Del Giudice G, Della Bianca V, et al: The neutrophil-activating protein (HP-NAP) of *Helicobacter pylori* is a protective antigen and a major virulence factor. *J Exp Med* 2000;191:1467-1476.

20.   Graham DY: The only good *Helicobacter pylori* is a dead *Helicobacter pylori*. *Lancet* 1997;350:70-71.

21.   Graham DY: Can therapy ever be denied for *Helicobacter pylori* infection? *Gastroenterology* 1997;113:S113-S117.

Index

A

acetylcysteine (Mucosil®)
106
achlorhydria 40
acid secretion 27, 32, 34,
35, 37, 38, 41-43, 49-51,
56, 98, 143, 148, 151
Aciphex® 98
acne rosacea 65
adhesin 28
alcohol 16
Alka-Seltzer® 98
ammonia 28, 75, 142, 178
amoxicillin 100-103, 105,
108-113, 115, 117, 120,
121, 166-169
anemia 89, 162
anorexia 89
antacids 50, 90, 97, 98,
105, 138
anticholinergic agents 99
antihistamines 103
antimicrobial therapy 97,
99, 112, 120, 128
antisecretory therapy 96,
98, 100, 114, 128, 129,
138, 141, 147
arthritis 63
aspirin 92
atrophic gastritis 51, 92

atrophic pangastritis 52,
55, 144, 145, 150
Avelox® 105
Axid® 98
azithromycin (Zithromax®)
102

B

Barrett's esophagus 56, 93,
138, 150, 153
Biaxin® 101, 102, 166, 167
biofilm phenomenon 119
bismuth 63, 77, 87, 100-
102, 107, 108, 111, 118-
121, 126, 167
bismuth subsalicylate
(Pepto-Bismol®) 100,
101, 111, 169
black stools 101, 121
BMT quadruple therapy
113
BMT triple therapy 107,
111-113, 120
BreathTek™ UBT 88

C

cag pathogenicity 29, 30,
149
CagA 29, 31, 176

I

IgA 78, 79, 175-178
IgA tests 78
IgG 77-79, 176
IgM 78, 79
income 16
indigestion 90
inoculum effect 118, 119
iron 40
iron deficiency anemia 162
ischemic heart disease 65
isocarboxazid (Marplan®)
   104

K

Koch's postulates 48, 49

L

lansoprazole (Prevacid®)
   98, 106, 110, 111, 113,
   166, 168
leukotrienes 32
Levaquin® 105
levofloxacin (Levaquin®)
   105, 120
lipopolysaccharide 30
lung cancer 49
lymphoma 7, 9, 40, 60-62,
   92, 125, 179

M

Maalox® 97
Maastricht consensus 64,
   109, 141

macrolides 103
Malakit 79
malnutrition 34
Marplan® 104
Meretek UBT Breath Test™
   (Meretek Diagnostics)
   84
metronidazole (Flagyl®,
   Protostat®) 63, 100-105,
   107, 108, 110-113, 116-
   121, 166-169
MicroVasive® 74
misoprostol (Cytotec®)
   99
molecular mimicry 59, 60
monoamine oxidase
   inhibitors 104, 114
moxifloxacin (Avelox®)
   105, 120
mucolytics 114
mucosa-associated
   lymphoid tissue
   (MALT) 42, 60-62, 92,
   125, 161
mucosal biopsy 71, 73-75,
   77, 87, 88, 124, 127,
   163
Mucosil® 106
Mycobutin® 105
Mylanta® 98

N

naproxen 63
Nardil™ 104
nasogastric tubes 22

NOTES

NOTES

NOTES